The Healthy Aging Book

CRAFTED BY SKRIUWER

Copyright © 2024 by Skriuwer.

All rights reserved. No part of this book may be used or reproduced in any form whatsoever without written permission except in the case of brief quotations in critical articles or reviews.

For more information, contact : **kontakt@skriuwer.com** (www.skriuwer.com)

TABLE OF CONTENTS

CHAPTER 1: UNDERSTANDING THE AGING PROCESS

- *Why the body changes over time and what it means for health*
- *Physical, mental, and social shifts that come with age*
- *Myths about getting older and how to handle concerns*

CHAPTER 2: GOOD NUTRITION & HEALTHY EATING HABITS

- *Balanced foods that fuel the body and mind*
- *Key nutrients older adults need and where to find them*
- *Meal-planning tips and mindful approaches to eating*

CHAPTER 3: THE IMPORTANCE OF DAILY MOVEMENT

- *How gentle exercises support heart, muscles, and bones*
- *Ways to include safe, simple physical activities at home*
- *Staying motivated when energy or mobility is limited*

CHAPTER 4: MAINTAINING A BALANCED WEIGHT

- *Why weight can shift with age and how it affects health*
- *Strategies for healthy weight management without extremes*
- *Practical tips to balance portions and stay active*

CHAPTER 5: HEART HEALTH AND BLOOD PRESSURE TIPS

- *Ways to protect your heart through daily habits*
- *Recognizing risks for high blood pressure and keeping it in check*
- *Easy lifestyle changes that aid circulation and lower strain*

CHAPTER 6: CARING FOR BONES AND JOINTS

- *How bones thin over time and methods to strengthen them*
- *Joint-friendly movements that reduce pain and stiffness*
- *Preventive steps to guard against fractures or injuries*

CHAPTER 7: SUPPORTING BRAIN HEALTH AND MEMORY

- *Why the mind changes with age and what you can do about it*
- *Brain-stimulating activities to keep thinking sharp*
- *Spotting early signs of memory concerns and handling them*

CHAPTER 8: EYE AND EAR CARE

- *Common vision and hearing changes in older adulthood*
- *Daily habits and check-ups that preserve these senses*
- *Tools and aids to adapt if eyesight or hearing declines*

CHAPTER 9: PROTECTING SKIN AND HAIR

- *Why skin and hair transform over time and simple care steps*
- *Preventing dryness, irritation, and minor infections*
- *Gentle approaches to hair thinning, graying, and scalp health*

CHAPTER 10: HANDLING STRESS IN OLDER AGE

- *Unique stress factors older adults may face*
- *Quick tricks to calm the mind and relax the body*
- *When to reach out for help if stress grows too high*

CHAPTER 11: SLEEP TIPS FOR BETTER REST

- *Reasons older adults experience changes in sleep*
- *Bedtime routines and environment tweaks to improve rest*
- *Overcoming common challenges like waking up too often*

CHAPTER 12: BUILDING STRONG SOCIAL TIES

- *Why positive relationships matter for emotional well-being*
- *Ideas for meeting new friends or reconnecting with family*
- *Social activities that nurture a sense of belonging*

CHAPTER 13: AVOIDING HARMFUL HABITS

- *How smoking, heavy drinking, or drug misuse affect older bodies*
- *Practical ways to cut back or quit dangerous behaviors*
- *Replacing harmful habits with healthier, more uplifting ones*

CHAPTER 14: KEEPING THE MIND ACTIVE AND SHARP

- *Lifelong learning and simple exercises to stay mentally engaged*
- *Creative hobbies that stimulate thought and reduce boredom*
- *Techniques for warding off forgetfulness and negative thinking*

CHAPTER 15: FINANCIAL & LEGAL BASICS FOR LATER LIFE

- *Organizing budgets, handling debts, and preparing for future costs*
- *Basic legal documents (wills, powers of attorney) to consider*
- *Protecting against scams or fraud targeted at older adults*

CHAPTER 16: PLANNING FOR RETIREMENT & WORK OPTIONS

- *Deciding when to retire and how to manage finances responsibly*
- *Flexible ways to keep working part-time or freelance*
- *Balancing free time, hobbies, and meaningful activities*

CHAPTER 17: EMOTIONAL HEALTH AND STAYING POSITIVE

- *Connecting emotions to well-being and handling grief or loss*
- *Building self-esteem through small achievements and caring mindset*
- *Seeking professional help if sadness or anxiety persist*

CHAPTER 18: GUARDING AGAINST COMMON ILLNESSES

- *Common infections and how to prevent them*
- *Maintaining cleanliness in daily habits and home environment*
- *Strengthening the immune system through vaccines and good hygiene*

CHAPTER 19: CHECK-UPS AND REGULAR SCREENINGS

- *Why routine appointments catch hidden problems early*
- *Key tests for heart, bones, cancer risks, and more*
- *Maximizing doctor visits with questions and preparation*

CHAPTER 20: CREATING A SAFE AND COMFORTABLE HOME

- *Adjusting entryways, floors, and furniture to reduce falls*
- *Making kitchens, bathrooms, and bedrooms more secure*
- *Using simple devices or technology for extra convenience and peace of mind*

CHAPTER 1: UNDERSTANDING THE AGING PROCESS

Aging is a normal part of life. It happens to everyone and everything. It is not a bad thing. It just means that as time goes by, our bodies go through changes. Some of these changes are easy to see, like when our hair turns gray. Other changes are hidden inside us, like how our hearts beat or how our bones feel. Learning about these changes can help us take better care of ourselves. It can also help us feel calmer about what lies ahead as we get older.

In this chapter, we will talk about what aging is and why it happens. We will look at how the body changes over time, including the way our muscles, bones, and organs might shift in how they work. We will also talk about changes in the mind, such as memory or mood. We will discuss how aging can affect our social lives, too. By understanding these different parts of aging, we can be prepared for what might happen and learn ways to stay as healthy as possible.

What Is Aging?

Aging means growing older. It is not just about how many birthdays you have had. It is about how your body and mind go through changes. When we talk about aging, we might think about wrinkles or gray hair. But that is only part of it. Aging also involves many things inside our bodies. Our hearts, lungs, bones, and brains all shift in different ways as we get older.

For some people, these changes begin earlier, and for others, they might happen later. It can also vary by genetics. That is, some families may see certain changes sooner or more often than other families. However, aging is not the same for everyone. Some individuals can stay strong and active for many years, while others might face health problems. Lifestyle can also play a big role. If someone eats well, exercises often, and avoids harmful habits, they may stay healthier than someone who does not.

Why Do People Age?

Scientists have studied aging for many years to figure out why it happens. There are many theories:

1. **Cell Damage Over Time**
   Our bodies are made up of tiny units called cells. Cells are always working to keep us going, like building blocks that do jobs in all our organs. Each day, cells face stress from normal wear and tear, pollution, sunlight, and other things. Over time, cells might stop working as well as they once did. This buildup of small changes can lead to aging.
2. **Genetics**
   Our genes are like instructions that tell our cells how to act. Some people have genes that help them stay healthier for a longer time. Others may have genes that make certain health problems more likely. Genes can also decide when certain signs of aging might show up.
3. **Hormones**
   Hormones are chemicals in our bodies that help control growth, metabolism, and many other functions. As we get older, our hormones might change. For example, women go through menopause, where their levels of certain hormones drop. This can lead to changes in bone health, mood, and other areas.
4. **Lifestyle Factors**
   What we eat, how often we move around, and how we handle stress can all impact the pace of aging. These factors can either help us feel better as we get older or speed up the effects of aging if we are not careful.

Aging is a mix of all these factors and more. It is complex, and there is no single cause that fits everyone. Instead, each body is different, and many elements combine to shape how we age.

Physical Changes During Aging

Many of the biggest changes in aging happen in the body. Some of these changes can be seen from the outside, but others are happening inside us. Here are some of the main physical changes that may occur as we grow older:

1. **Bones and Joints**
   - **Bone Density**: Our bones are strong, but they can become thinner with age. Thinner bones are weaker bones. This can lead to problems like fractures or osteoporosis.
   - **Joints**: Joints are the places where bones connect, such as knees, hips, and shoulders. With age, the protective covering in our joints

can wear down, making it harder to move. This can lead to stiffness or pain.
    - **What to Do**: Staying active can keep bones and joints healthier. Some simple exercises, like walking, can be good for bone strength. Making sure to eat foods with calcium and vitamin D can also help maintain bone health.
2. **Muscles and Strength**
    - **Muscle Mass**: As we age, we might lose some muscle mass. Muscles can become weaker if we do not use them.
    - **Flexibility**: We might find it harder to bend or stretch. Keeping up with gentle daily stretches can help maintain flexibility.
    - **What to Do**: Strength exercises, like lifting light weights or using resistance bands, can help keep muscles strong. Even everyday tasks like carrying groceries can make a difference.
3. **Heart and Blood Vessels**
    - **Heart Health**: The heart can become less flexible with age. The walls of blood vessels might get stiffer, too. This can lead to higher blood pressure or other problems if not cared for.
    - **Changes in Blood Flow**: Blood flow might slow down, which can lead to feeling cold more often or healing from cuts and bruises more slowly.
    - **What to Do**: Regular check-ups can help spot issues early. Activities like walking and swimming can keep the heart strong. Eating heart-friendly foods, such as fruits, vegetables, whole grains, and lean proteins, also helps.
4. **Lungs and Breathing**
    - **Lung Capacity**: Our lungs can hold less air as we get older. This is why some people feel out of breath sooner than they used to.
    - **Changes in Airway**: The muscles that help us breathe might get weaker, making it harder to take deep breaths.
    - **What to Do**: Light aerobic activity like brisk walking or gentle cycling can help keep the lungs stronger. Practicing deep-breathing exercises can also support better lung function.
5. **Digestive System**
    - **Slower Digestion**: The digestive process can slow down. This might lead to problems like constipation or bloating.
    - **Changes in Nutrient Absorption**: Our bodies might have a harder time absorbing certain vitamins, like vitamin B12.

- **What to Do**: Eating more fiber can help, as well as drinking enough water. If you notice ongoing digestive issues, checking with a doctor can be a good idea.
6. **Skin, Hair, and Nails**
    - **Skin**: Skin might become thinner, drier, and less stretchy. Wrinkles often appear. Cuts and bruises might take longer to heal.
    - **Hair**: Hair might turn gray or white. It can also become thinner.
    - **Nails**: Nails can grow more slowly and become brittle.
    - **What to Do**: Keeping skin clean, using mild moisturizers, and avoiding too much direct sun can help. A balanced diet also supports healthy hair and nails.
7. **Hormonal Changes**
    - **Menopause**: In women, menopause can cause changes in monthly cycles, mood, sleep, and bone health due to shifts in hormone levels.
    - **Men's Hormones**: Some men might see changes in energy level or mood over time, possibly related to slow changes in certain hormones.
    - **What to Do**: Talking with a doctor can help guide you through these changes. Making lifestyle adjustments, such as healthy eating and regular exercise, can reduce some of the effects.

All these physical changes are part of getting older. They do not happen all at once. Some might appear sooner, while others may come later. It is important to remember that everyone is unique. You might face some changes more than others. By staying aware of these common shifts, you can take steps to stay healthy and feel better for longer.

Mental and Emotional Changes

Aging is not just about the body. The mind also goes through changes. Some of these changes can be positive, like becoming wiser or better at handling problems. Other changes might be more challenging, such as memory slips or mood shifts. Here are some areas to keep in mind:

1. **Memory and Thinking**
    - **Recall**: Many people find that they might forget small details more easily than before. For example, forgetting where the car keys are or missing an appointment.

- **Processing Speed**: It might take longer to handle new information. Learning something new can feel slower.
- **Staying Sharp**: Keeping the mind active by reading, doing simple puzzles, or chatting with friends can help the brain stay strong. If memory problems become serious, it is best to visit a doctor.

2. **Emotional Health**
   - **Changes in Mood**: Some older adults might feel sadness or worry more often than they did when they were younger. This can happen because of hormonal changes, life events, or health problems.
   - **Losses and Grief**: Aging can sometimes bring moments of loss, such as losing loved ones. Grief and sadness can affect emotional health.
   - **Seeking Help**: Talking with trusted friends, family, or a counselor can help. Staying connected with others can lessen sadness and support emotional balance.

3. **Self-Confidence**
   - **Body Image**: Changes in appearance might lead some people to feel less confident. They may worry about wrinkles or weight.
   - **Skills and Abilities**: If someone can no longer move around the way they used to, they might feel frustrated.
   - **Building Confidence**: Setting simple goals and focusing on what you can do, rather than what you cannot, can help. Finding new hobbies or connecting with friends can boost morale.

4. **Stress and Coping**
   - **Life Changes**: Some people retire, move to a smaller home, or see family members move away. These changes can be stressful.
   - **Coping Methods**: Easy techniques like breathing exercises or speaking with a supportive person can help calm stress.
   - **Professional Support**: If stress becomes overwhelming, a mental health professional or a doctor can provide guidance and strategies.

Everyone's mental and emotional experience is different, but many older adults face some of these situations. It is helpful to be prepared and to seek help if something feels too hard. That way, you can keep your mind and emotions in a healthier place.

Social and Relationship Changes

Aging can also affect relationships and social life. Here are some ways people might notice shifts:

1. **Spending Time with Others**
    - **Social Circles**: As people get older, their group of friends may change. Some friends might move away to live closer to their kids. Others might face health problems that keep them indoors. This can shrink social circles.
    - **Staying Connected**: Attending community events or reaching out by phone can help. Even short calls can brighten a day.
2. **Family Dynamics**
    - **Adult Children**: Children might be grown and have their own families. Some older adults might see their grown children less often.
    - **Grandchildren**: For some, grandchildren can bring joy and fresh energy. But there can also be challenges if older adults are asked to help with babysitting more often than they want.
    - **Keeping Boundaries**: Talking openly about needs and limits can help maintain good relationships with adult children and other family members.
3. **Loss of Loved Ones**
    - **Grieving**: As time goes on, older adults might lose close friends or a partner. Grief can be hard to handle, and it often leads to loneliness.
    - **Finding Support**: Support groups or online communities can help someone feel less alone in grief. Talking with a professional can also be valuable.
4. **New Roles**
    - **Retirement**: Leaving a job after many years can be a big change. Some people enjoy the free time, while others miss the routine of work.
    - **Volunteering or Community Work**: Some older adults find purpose by helping in local groups, libraries, or schools. This can fill the space that work once occupied.

Social changes are normal with aging. Even though some can feel challenging, there are ways to find support and stay connected. Knowing that these shifts can happen makes them easier to handle.

Common Myths About Aging

There are many ideas about getting older that may not be true. Here are a few common myths:

1. **Myth**: "Older people are always sick."
   Truth: While some older adults do face health problems, many are still active. The way we live and our genes both affect how healthy we stay.
2. **Myth**: "It is too late to get fit."
   Truth: Regular activity helps at any age. Even gentle walks can improve balance and strength, no matter how old someone is.
3. **Myth**: "Older adults do not learn new things."
   Truth: People can continue to learn and grow mentally. It might take a bit more time to pick up new skills, but the mind can stay active.
4. **Myth**: "Loneliness is just part of getting old."
   Truth: Feeling lonely is not something that has to happen. Reaching out to friends, family, or community groups can help keep social connections strong.

Correcting these myths can help us have a more positive view of aging. It also shows that getting older can come with many possibilities if we take care of ourselves and remain open to trying new ways of living.

Ways to Support the Body and Mind

Understanding what is happening with aging can help us decide what to do about it. Here are some basic ways to stay healthier and stronger:

1. **Regular Check-Ups**
   - Seeing a doctor for yearly check-ups can catch health issues early.
   - Regular dental and eye exams are also important.
   - Blood tests and other screenings can make sure you stay on top of any concerns.
2. **Healthy Eating**
   - Focus on fruits, vegetables, lean proteins, whole grains, and dairy (or dairy substitutes if needed).
   - Limit foods high in sugar or unhealthy fats.
   - Staying hydrated by drinking plenty of water can help with digestion and overall well-being.

3. **Staying Active**
   - Even simple exercises, like walks or gentle stretching, can help keep muscles and bones strong.
   - Some people enjoy group classes, like water aerobics, which can be good for joints.
4. **Staying Mentally Engaged**
   - Puzzles, reading, or trying to learn simple new skills can keep the mind active.
   - Talking with others about ideas or current events can also stimulate thinking.
5. **Managing Stress**
   - Easy breathing exercises or spending quiet time in a peaceful place can reduce stress.
   - Sharing feelings with trusted friends or family can also help you feel better.
6. **Getting Enough Sleep**
   - Aim for about seven to nine hours of sleep a night, if possible.
   - A calm bedtime routine, like reading or listening to soft music, can improve rest.

These basic ideas might seem simple, but they can make a huge difference in how we feel as we age. Taking steps to care for our bodies and minds gives us a better chance of feeling well for longer.

Looking Ahead

Aging is something that happens to all of us, but we can still guide many parts of our well-being. By learning about the common changes in our bodies, minds, and social lives, we can be prepared to handle them. We might not be able to stop every change, but we can do our best to keep them from causing too many problems.

In the coming chapters, we will talk more about ways to stay healthy, including taking care of our hearts, bones, and brains. We will also talk about handling stress and getting enough rest. We will look at social factors, too, because having good relationships can help us stay happier and healthier.

Though aging can bring challenges, there are plenty of steps we can take to feel our best. Staying informed is the first step. By being aware, we can make smart choices and keep ourselves on the path to better health.

That is the key to understanding aging: it is not something to fear, but a stage of life that we can prepare for. When we know what to look out for, we can take action that helps us feel more in control. Learning about these topics now can lead to many better days ahead.

CHAPTER 2: GOOD NUTRITION AND HEALTHY EATING HABITS

What we eat plays a big role in our health, especially as we get older. A balanced diet gives our bodies the vitamins, minerals, and other nutrients we need to function well. It can help us keep a healthy weight, have more energy, and avoid some health issues. However, as we age, our nutritional needs might change. Our bodies might need more of some vitamins or less of certain foods to stay healthy.

In this chapter, we will talk about what kinds of foods are good for older adults. We will discuss the different food groups and how they help the body. We will also talk about why we need certain nutrients more as we age, like calcium or protein. We will share tips on how to plan meals, shop for groceries, and prepare simple, healthy dishes. All these pointers can help you or a loved one eat better for strong health and better well-being.

The Basics of a Balanced Diet

A balanced diet means eating a mix of foods that give us different kinds of nutrients. Each food group serves a purpose. Here are some main groups and why they matter:

1. **Fruits and Vegetables**
    - **Importance**: Fruits and vegetables are full of vitamins, minerals, and fiber. They can help keep our hearts healthy and support our immune systems.
    - **Variety**: Different colors mean different nutrients. For example, orange vegetables like carrots or sweet potatoes have beta-carotene, while green vegetables like spinach have vitamin K.
    - **Tips**: Try to include a fruit or vegetable at every meal. Frozen or canned options can also be healthy if they have no added sugar or salt.
2. **Whole Grains**
    - **Examples**: Whole wheat bread, brown rice, oats, barley.
    - **Importance**: Whole grains give us energy, fiber, and vitamins like B vitamins. They can help control blood sugar and keep us feeling full longer.

- **Tips**: Choose whole grain products whenever possible. Look for labels that say "100% whole grain" or "whole wheat."
3. **Lean Proteins**
    - **Examples**: Skinless chicken, fish, beans, lentils, tofu, eggs.
    - **Importance**: Protein helps build and maintain muscle and other tissues in the body. It also helps with hormone and enzyme production.
    - **Tips**: Include a source of protein at every meal. If you eat meat, try to choose lean cuts or fish rich in healthy fats like salmon. If you prefer vegetarian choices, beans and lentils are great.
4. **Dairy or Dairy Alternatives**
    - **Examples**: Low-fat milk, cheese, yogurt, soy milk, almond milk with added calcium.
    - **Importance**: Dairy provides calcium, vitamin D, and protein. These are especially important for bones.
    - **Tips**: Some people have a hard time digesting dairy. Alternatives with added calcium and vitamin D can help.
5. **Healthy Fats**
    - **Examples**: Avocados, nuts, seeds, olive oil, fatty fish like salmon.
    - **Importance**: Fats are needed for hormone production, cell health, and energy. But the type of fat matters. Unsaturated fats (from plants and fish) are better than saturated fats (from butter or fatty meats).
    - **Tips**: Replace butter with olive oil when possible. Use nuts as a snack instead of chips.

When we eat a range of foods from these groups, we get the nutrients we need. It is also good to limit things like sugary snacks or drinks, fried foods, and processed foods. These can be okay in small amounts, but too many can affect health over time.

Special Nutrient Needs in Older Age

As we age, our bodies need certain nutrients more than before. Some of these nutrients include:

1. **Calcium and Vitamin D**
    - **Reason**: These nutrients keep bones strong. As bones can thin out with age, getting enough calcium and vitamin D is extra important.

- **Sources**: Dairy products, fortified cereals, leafy greens, fish like sardines or salmon, and sunlight (for vitamin D).
- **Tip**: Check with a doctor about blood levels of vitamin D. Supplements might be needed if levels are low.

2. **Protein**
   - **Reason**: Protein helps maintain muscle mass, which can weaken over time.
   - **Sources**: Chicken, fish, beans, eggs, tofu, and lean meats.
   - **Tip**: Spread protein throughout the day. Have a source of protein at breakfast, lunch, and dinner.

3. **Fiber**
   - **Reason**: Helps with digestion and can lower the chance of heart problems.
   - **Sources**: Whole grains, fruits, vegetables, beans, and nuts.
   - **Tip**: Increase fiber slowly if you are not used to it, and drink enough water to help fiber do its job.

4. **B Vitamins**
   - **Reason**: Certain B vitamins, like B12, help the body make red blood cells and support brain function. As we age, the body might absorb less vitamin B12.
   - **Sources**: Meat, fish, eggs, dairy, and fortified cereals.
   - **Tip**: Ask a doctor for a blood test to check levels if you feel tired or weak.

5. **Antioxidants**
   - **Reason**: These help fight damage caused by stress and the environment. They can support overall health, including eye and heart health.
   - **Sources**: Brightly colored fruits and vegetables (berries, carrots, spinach), nuts, and seeds.
   - **Tip**: The best approach is to eat a variety of colorful fruits and vegetables.

Sometimes, it can be hard to get enough of these nutrients from food alone. In those cases, a doctor might suggest supplements. But it is best to get as many nutrients as possible from whole foods.

Tips for Meal Planning

Planning meals can help ensure that you get the right mix of nutrients each day. Here are some simple steps:

1. **Plan Ahead**
    - Write down meals for the week.
    - Make a shopping list that includes all the foods you need.
2. **Balanced Plates**
    - Aim to fill half your plate with vegetables.
    - Fill a quarter of your plate with protein.
    - Fill the last quarter with whole grains.
    - Add a serving of fruit or dairy on the side if you like.
3. **Consider Your Schedule**
    - If you are busy at certain times, plan quick meals like sandwiches on whole grain bread with lean protein.
    - If you have more free time on other days, cook bigger batches of soup or stew, and freeze some for later.
4. **Use Leftovers**
    - Cook extra so you have some for another meal.
    - Try to store leftovers in single servings so they are easy to heat up.
    - Label and date them in the fridge or freezer.
5. **Mix It Up**
    - Include different types of fruits, vegetables, proteins, and grains so you do not get bored.
    - Vary cooking methods (baking, grilling, steaming) to keep meals interesting.

When meals are planned out, it becomes easier to follow a healthy eating pattern. This also reduces waste and saves money because you only buy what you need.

Grocery Shopping for Healthy Eating

Going to the store with a plan helps you stick to healthy choices. Here are some tips:

1. **Shop the Perimeter**

- Most stores place produce, dairy, meat, and fish around the outer edges. These are often the healthiest sections.
- Be careful in the aisles in the middle, which hold many processed foods.

2. **Read Labels**
    - Look for foods that have fewer added sugars and fewer ingredients you do not recognize.
    - Check the sodium (salt) content, especially in canned goods or packaged meals.
3. **Buy in Season**
    - Fruits and vegetables are cheaper and taste better when they are in season.
    - If what you want is not in season, consider frozen produce, which can still have plenty of nutrients.
4. **Avoid Shopping While Hungry**
    - If you go shopping while you are very hungry, you might grab snacks or sweets that are not on your list.
    - Eat a small meal or a healthy snack before heading to the store.
5. **Look for Sales and Deals**
    - Healthy eating does not have to cost a lot. Watch for sales on lean meats, whole grains, and fresh produce.
    - Store brands can be cheaper than name brands and still have the same nutrition.

By thinking about your shopping before you step into the store, you can make better choices and avoid bringing home items that might not support your health.

Simple Cooking Methods

Cooking healthy meals does not have to be hard or time-consuming. Here are some easy ways to cook:

1. **Baking or Roasting**
    - Ideal for vegetables, chicken, or fish.
    - Add a little olive oil and simple spices for flavor.
    - Cook in the oven until the food is tender and lightly browned.
2. **Steaming**
    - Great for vegetables like broccoli, carrots, or green beans.

- Keeps many of the vitamins in the food.
- Use a steamer basket or a small amount of water in a pot.
3. **Grilling**
   - Works well for fish, chicken, or vegetables like zucchini.
   - Use low-sodium seasoning or lemon juice for extra taste.
   - If using an outdoor grill, make sure foods are cooked safely.
4. **Stir-Frying**
   - Quick method for lean meats and lots of chopped vegetables.
   - Use a small amount of healthy oil, like olive oil.
   - Add low-sodium soy sauce or spices for flavor.
5. **Slow Cooking**
   - Perfect for stews or soups with beans, vegetables, and lean meats.
   - It can cook for hours without needing attention.
   - Make enough for multiple meals and freeze the extras.
6. **Microwaving**
   - Handy for heating up leftovers or cooking small amounts of veggies.
   - Cover the food lightly to keep moisture in.
   - Check the food halfway to stir or move items around for even cooking.

By focusing on these basic methods, you can create meals that are flavorful and nutritious without spending too much time in the kitchen. Also, these methods use less oil and can help cut back on extra calories.

Healthy Snacking

Snacks can be part of a healthy diet if chosen wisely. Here are some good snack ideas:

1. **Fruit**
   - Fresh fruits like apple slices, grapes, or berries are sweet and contain fiber.
   - Pair apple slices with a small spoon of peanut butter for extra protein.
2. **Yogurt**
   - Low-fat or Greek yogurt provides protein and calcium.
   - Top it with some fresh fruit or a sprinkle of nuts.
3. **Nuts and Seeds**

- Almonds, walnuts, sunflower seeds, or pumpkin seeds have healthy fats and protein.
- Watch portion sizes because they can be high in calories.
4. **Vegetables**
    - Carrot sticks, cucumber slices, or bell pepper strips can be dipped in hummus.
    - Celery sticks with peanut butter add some crunch.
5. **Whole Grain Crackers**
    - Look for crackers made with whole wheat or other whole grains.
    - Top them with a slice of cheese or turkey for a quick protein boost.

Snacks can help keep energy levels steady, but be aware of how many snacks you eat in a day. It is easy to eat too many calories if you are not careful. Focus on snacks that offer nutrition, not just empty calories.

Hydration and Beverages

Drinking enough water is just as important as eating well. Dehydration can cause tiredness, dizziness, and other problems. As people age, they might not feel thirsty as often, so they must remember to drink fluids regularly.

1. **Water**
    - Best choice for staying hydrated.
    - If you do not like plain water, add slices of lemon, cucumber, or berries for flavor.
2. **Herbal Tea**
    - Teas like chamomile, peppermint, or rooibos can be soothing and free of caffeine.
    - Drink them hot or cold without adding too much sugar or sweetener.
3. **Low-Fat Milk or Dairy Alternatives**
    - Provides nutrients like calcium and vitamin D.
    - Watch out for added sugars in flavored milk or milk alternatives.
4. **Limit Sugary Drinks**
    - Sodas and fruit juices with added sugar can lead to weight gain and other issues.
    - If you like juice, choose 100% juice and stick to small servings.
5. **Limit Alcohol**

- Too much alcohol can harm organs and lead to falls or accidents.
- Talk to your doctor about safe amounts if you choose to drink.

Keeping a bottle of water nearby can remind you to sip throughout the day. If you notice signs of dehydration, like dry mouth or dark-colored urine, try to drink more water.

Overcoming Common Eating Challenges

Some older adults find it harder to eat well due to certain challenges:

1. **Reduced Appetite**
   - **Cause**: Could be related to medications or health problems.
   - **Solution**: Eat small, nutrient-rich meals more often. Try to include high-protein snacks like yogurt or cheese.
2. **Difficulty Chewing or Swallowing**
   - **Cause**: Dental issues or throat problems.
   - **Solution**: Choose softer foods like oatmeal, mashed vegetables, or soups. Cook vegetables until they are tender.
3. **Changes in Taste and Smell**
   - **Cause**: Medications or simply the effects of aging.
   - **Solution**: Use herbs and spices to add flavor. Try new recipes that use different seasonings.
4. **Food Budget**
   - **Cause**: People on a fixed income might worry about the cost of food.
   - **Solution**: Buy items on sale and choose cost-effective proteins like beans or eggs. Frozen fruits and vegetables are often cheaper and last longer.
5. **Eating Alone**
   - **Cause**: Some older adults live by themselves, making mealtimes lonely.
   - **Solution**: Invite a friend over or arrange meal gatherings at senior centers if possible. Sometimes, even talking on the phone during a meal can help.

It is important to note that if you face any of these problems, speaking with a healthcare professional or a nutritionist might help. They can offer personalized advice.

Putting It All Together

Eating well does not have to be stressful. Here is an example of what a day of healthy eating could look like:

- **Breakfast**:
    - Oatmeal topped with berries and a splash of low-fat milk
    - A boiled egg on the side
    - A glass of water or herbal tea
- **Mid-Morning Snack**:
    - Apple slices with a spoon of peanut butter
- **Lunch**:
    - A green salad with chopped vegetables (cucumber, tomato, bell pepper) and a lean protein like grilled chicken
    - Whole grain bread slice on the side
    - Water with a slice of lemon
- **Afternoon Snack**:
    - Low-fat yogurt with a sprinkle of nuts
- **Dinner**:
    - Baked fish (like salmon or tilapia) with a squeeze of lemon juice
    - Steamed broccoli and carrots
    - Brown rice
    - Water or low-fat milk
- **Evening Snack** (optional):
    - Whole grain crackers with low-fat cheese
    - Herbal tea, unsweetened

This plan includes a good balance of proteins, whole grains, fruits, vegetables, and dairy. Adjust portion sizes based on your needs. The idea is to show how different foods can fit together in a day to provide all-around nutrition.

CHAPTER 3: THE IMPORTANCE OF DAILY MOVEMENT

Staying active can help us feel better and support many parts of our health. Daily movement does not always mean heavy workouts or running marathons. It can be gentle actions that keep our bodies in motion, like short walks or simple chores. Small activities each day add up to help our hearts, muscles, bones, and even our mood. In this chapter, we will look at why daily movement is useful, how it helps different parts of our well-being, and how older adults can include more physical activity in their lives without putting themselves at risk.

What Does Daily Movement Mean?

Daily movement can mean many things. It can be a short walk to the mailbox, a gentle dance to music, or even basic tasks like washing dishes. The main idea is to avoid sitting for too long and to move our bodies in a safe way that matches our abilities. Each person will have a different level of activity that feels comfortable. For some, daily movement might include a slow stroll in the park. Others might enjoy more active pastimes, like swimming or light gardening. The goal is to keep blood flowing and muscles working.

The reason we focus on "daily" movement, rather than once a week, is because the body benefits from regular use. Muscles, bones, and joints grow more used to mild stress if we move a bit each day. This can lead to better strength over time. Many small sessions of activity can give just as many benefits as one long session, especially for those who have a hard time doing long periods of exercise.

How Does Daily Movement Help the Body?

1. **Heart and Circulation**
   - **Improved Blood Flow**: When we move, the heart pumps blood more actively. This means more oxygen goes to the muscles and organs. Over time, this can help lower the risk of heart problems.

- **Stable Blood Pressure**: Regular activity can help keep blood pressure in a healthier range. It might also help if blood pressure is already high.
2. **Muscles**
    - **Strength and Tone**: Daily actions like walking or light lifting keep muscles active. This can slow the loss of muscle mass that can happen with aging.
    - **Balance and Stability**: Stronger muscles can help older adults stay steady on their feet, lowering the chance of falls.
3. **Bones**
    - **Bone Strength**: Bones are living tissues that respond to activity. Gentle stress from movement, such as walking or going up stairs, can help keep bones stronger.
    - **Joint Flexibility**: Joints can become stiff when not used often. Daily movement can help keep them flexible and less painful.
4. **Weight Control**
    - **Burning Calories**: Being active helps use up more energy, which can support a healthier weight. Even modest increases in movement can make a difference.
    - **Boosting Metabolism**: The body might keep burning some extra calories even after an activity session ends, especially if there is some muscle involvement.
5. **Body Functions**
    - **Digestion**: Light movement can assist with digestion by stimulating the body's processes.
    - **Immune System**: Some studies suggest that regular activity supports the immune system, making it easier for the body to handle minor illnesses.

Daily movement, in short, supports many functions. It is a simple way to keep the body working better for longer.

Benefits for the Mind

It is not just the body that gains from daily movement. The mind can also benefit in a few ways:

1. **Mood Improvement**

- Moving releases certain chemicals in the brain that can lead to a more positive feeling.
- Activities can also be fun or social, which lifts spirits.
2. **Sharper Thinking**
    - Regular movement might help with thinking skills. Some research suggests that physical activity can improve attention and memory tasks.
    - Learning new movements or routines (like dance steps) can challenge the brain in a good way.
3. **Stress Relief**
    - Taking a short walk outside or doing a gentle stretch can help clear the mind and reduce tension.
    - Regular activity has been linked to lower stress levels over time.

Even mild actions, such as moving the arms while seated, can give small boosts to how we feel. This can be especially helpful if someone is dealing with sadness or worry.

Types of Daily Movement

Daily movement does not have to be the same each day. Here are some ideas:

1. **Walking**
    - One of the easiest ways to move more. People can do it almost anywhere.
    - Walking can be adjusted to fit different fitness levels. Strolling slowly for five minutes might be enough for some, while others might walk faster or go for a longer period.
2. **Household Tasks**
    - Doing the laundry, vacuuming, or sweeping floors counts as activity.
    - Yard work, such as raking leaves or light gardening, can also raise the heart rate gently.
3. **Chair Exercises**
    - Some people have trouble standing or walking for long. Seated exercises can still work the muscles.
    - Simple arm raises with light weights or leg lifts while seated can help maintain strength.
4. **Stretching and Flexibility Work**

- Stretching daily can help ease stiffness in joints and muscles.
- Can be done after waking up or before bedtime to relax the body.
5. **Low-Impact Aerobics**
    - Activities like water aerobics or gentle dancing are good for those who have joint concerns.
    - The water helps support the body, lowering stress on knees and hips.
6. **Balance Activities**
    - Practicing to stand on one foot (with support nearby) or walking heel-to-toe in a straight line can improve balance.
    - Some people find simple balance routines helpful for lowering the risk of falling.

Each type of movement can help in different ways. It is fine to try many and choose the ones that feel most comfortable or enjoyable.

How Often Should We Move?

In many cases, health experts recommend at least a small amount of movement daily. Even ten minutes at a time is helpful. Some guidelines suggest aiming for about 30 minutes of mild to moderate activity most days, but this can vary based on each person's health and doctor's advice.

For those who cannot do 30 minutes in one go, splitting it into three short sessions of 10 minutes throughout the day can still help. For instance, a quick walk in the morning, some gentle stretching in the afternoon, and another short walk after dinner could reach that total. The key is making sure that the activity feels safe and is matched to the person's ability level.

Staying Safe While Moving

Older adults might have special concerns, such as balance problems, joint pain, or health conditions like heart disease. Here are tips to stay safe:

1. **Check with a Doctor**
    - If someone has a health issue, it is wise to ask a medical professional what forms of movement are best.

- A doctor can also suggest whether certain movements should be avoided.
2. **Wear the Right Shoes**
   - Footwear that fits properly and has good support can lower the chance of slipping.
   - If walking outside, look for shoes with non-slip soles.
3. **Start Slowly**
   - If the body is not used to regular activity, do short sessions first.
   - Increase the time or intensity bit by bit if it feels okay.
4. **Stay Hydrated**
   - Have water before, during, and after any movement session if needed.
   - Even mild movement can make us lose some fluids.
5. **Warm Up and Cool Down**
   - Begin each activity with a gentle warm-up, such as slow marching in place, to prepare the body.
   - End with easy stretches to help muscles relax.
6. **Watch for Pain**
   - Feeling some tiredness is normal, but sharp pain is a sign to stop.
   - If pain does not go away, talk with a doctor.
7. **Be Aware of Surroundings**
   - Choose flat surfaces that are clear of objects that could trip you.
   - When trying new outdoor routes, go with a friend or let someone know where you are going.

These steps can help make daily movement safer and more comfortable.

Bringing Movement into Everyday Life

Sometimes older adults worry that they do not have the time or energy for formal exercise sessions. But daily movement can fit into routines in small ways. Here are some simple methods to move more:

1. **Short Walk Breaks**
   - Every hour or so, stand up and walk around the house or yard for a couple of minutes.
   - If you are watching TV, use commercial breaks as a reminder to stand up and stretch.
2. **Stand While Doing Tasks**

- If you are reading the mail or talking on the phone, do it while standing if possible.
- This adds a bit of movement throughout the day.

3. **Use the Stairs**
    - If stairs are safe for you, going up a few steps can provide a gentle boost for leg muscles.
    - Take it slow and hold on to a handrail if needed.
4. **Park Further Away**
    - When heading to a store or appointment, park a little farther from the door (if you drive).
    - This increases the number of steps you take.
5. **Household Chores**
    - Doing your own chores, like washing dishes, making the bed, or sweeping, adds mild movement.
    - Turn on some music to make it more pleasant.
6. **Simple Strength Exercises**
    - Keep light hand weights or small water bottles around. Use them for short sets of bicep curls during the day.
    - If you use a stable chair, try slow and careful sit-to-stand movements.

All of these actions can become part of a regular habit, helping keep the body active without needing a special workout space or long blocks of free time.

Dealing with Motivation Problems

Sometimes people know that movement is good for them, but they still find it hard to get started. Here are some suggestions:

1. **Set Easy Goals**
    - Instead of aiming for 30 minutes right away, start with a five-minute walk or a few leg lifts.
    - Celebrate reaching small steps without using the word "celebrate." Instead, acknowledge the progress and let yourself feel satisfied that you reached your own target.
2. **Find a Buddy**
    - Ask a friend or family member to join you. Doing things together can make it more enjoyable and keep you accountable.

- If no one nearby can join, consider making phone calls to check in with each other about daily activity.
3. **Pick Something Enjoyable**
   - Some people like dancing, others prefer gardening. Some enjoy simple tasks like tidying up to music.
   - When an activity feels good or fun, it is easier to keep doing it.
4. **Track Progress**
   - Keep a simple notebook where you write down what you did each day.
   - Seeing a list of your accomplishments can be encouraging.
5. **Be Kind to Yourself**
   - If you skip a day, that is okay. Try to move again the next day.
   - Focus on improvements in how you feel rather than trying to be perfect.

Moving with Limited Mobility

Not everyone can walk easily or stand for long. People with limited mobility can still find ways to move safely:

1. **Chair Aerobics**
   - Sit in a sturdy chair and move your arms and legs to music.
   - Lift your arms overhead and then bring them down, or move your legs in a marching motion.
   - This can raise the heart rate a bit without stressing the joints.
2. **Seated Strength Work**
   - Use small weights or resistance bands while seated to build muscle in the arms and upper body.
   - Keep movements slow and controlled.
3. **Gentle Arm and Leg Movements in Bed**
   - For those who are mostly in bed, even small lifts of arms or legs can help blood flow.
   - A caregiver or family member can assist with slow, gentle range-of-motion activities.
4. **Stretching**
   - Stretch arms, neck, and legs from a seated position to keep them from feeling stiff.
   - Do not force any movement if it hurts.

Adapting daily movement to what is possible is important. Even mild movements can have positive effects on circulation and mood.

Building Strength Over Time

As we grow older, we may lose some strength naturally, but that does not mean we cannot maintain or improve the muscle we still have. Light strength exercises can help:

1. **Bodyweight Exercises**
   - Modified squats (holding on to a chair), heel raises, and push-ups against a wall can build muscle.
   - Start with very few reps (like five) and add more if it feels okay.
2. **Resistance Bands**
   - These stretchy bands can be used for arm curls, shoulder presses, and more. They come in different thickness levels.
   - Always begin with a band that gives mild resistance, and move slowly.
3. **Light Weights**
   - Hand weights can help strengthen arms and shoulders.
   - Start with 1 or 2 pounds if needed, and do a small number of reps.

Regular strength exercises, done two or three times a week, can make daily tasks easier, such as lifting groceries or climbing stairs.

The Role of Balance and Flexibility

Older adults often worry about falling. Keeping the body flexible and steady helps lower that risk:

1. **Flexibility**
   - Muscles and tendons can become tight, which might make movement harder.
   - Simple daily stretches, like touching your toes (if comfortable) or gently reaching overhead, can loosen tight spots.
2. **Balance**

- Practice standing on one foot for a few seconds while holding a sturdy surface.
- Walk slowly in a straight line, putting one foot right in front of the other.
- Sit and stand from a chair without using your hands if that feels safe.

Working on balance can bring greater confidence when walking and doing normal tasks. Flexibility also helps with reaching for items and bending down carefully.

Signs You Are Doing Well

If you move regularly, you might notice:

1. **More Energy**
   - Even a small increase in movement can make daily tasks feel less tiring.
   - You might feel more awake during the day.
2. **Less Stiffness**
   - Joints may not feel as stiff, especially after sitting for long periods.
   - Muscles might recover faster after light activities.
3. **Better Mood**
   - People often report feeling lighter and more at ease after doing mild exercise or stretching.
   - Worries might seem a bit easier to handle.
4. **Stable Weight**
   - You could notice some weight benefits if you combine regular movement with wise eating habits.
   - Clothes might fit better or you might see small changes in how you look.

If you do not notice changes right away, do not feel discouraged. A few days of movement might not show major results, but over weeks or months, the benefits often become clearer.

Handling Challenges

Life can throw obstacles in our path, such as minor illnesses or busy schedules. Here are ways to keep daily movement going:

1. **Illness or Injury**
    - If you feel sick, it might be wise to rest. But once you feel better, try gentle movements to help the body recover.
    - If a specific injury bothers you, talk with a doctor or physical therapist about activities that are safe.
2. **Bad Weather**
    - If it is too cold, hot, or wet outside, move indoors. You can walk around the house, use a hallway, or follow a simple indoor routine.
    - If you have space, you might keep an exercise DVD or online video handy.
3. **Busy Schedule**
    - Fit short movement breaks in between tasks. Even a few minutes here and there can add up.
    - Combine tasks with activity, such as tidying the living room while you chat on the phone.
4. **Changing Abilities**
    - If you find that certain movements become too hard, switch to something gentler.
    - Seek out a physical therapist if you need a tailored plan.

Staying flexible with your approach can help you keep moving even when things are not perfect.

When to Seek Help

Sometimes people feel worried about getting hurt or making a health problem worse. If you are not sure what kinds of movement are best, consider these steps:

1. **Ask Your Doctor**
    - Bring a list of what you want to try, and see if there are any warnings.
    - Ask for a referral to a physical therapist if needed.
2. **Join a Group Class**

- Some community centers or local groups offer classes for seniors that focus on gentle stretches or light aerobics.
- An instructor can guide you on proper form so you do not strain a muscle.
3. **Family and Friends**
    - If you have trouble getting around on your own, a friend or family member might help by walking with you or driving you to a park.
    - Support from loved ones can make activity feel safer and less lonely.

If you ever feel sharp pain, dizziness, or sudden weakness during movement, pause and consult a medical professional. Safety should come first.

Simple Moves to Try at Home

Below are a few examples of moves you can do in a safe area. Remember to warm up first and move slowly:

1. **Seated Leg Extensions**
    - Sit in a sturdy chair.
    - Extend one leg out in front, hold for a moment, then lower it.
    - Repeat on the other side. This works leg muscles without putting weight on joints.
2. **Chair Squats**
    - Stand in front of a chair with your feet shoulder-width apart.
    - Slowly bend your knees and lower your body as if to sit, then stand back up before you fully sit down.
    - Keep a hand on the chair's armrest if needed.
3. **Arm Circles**
    - Stand or sit with arms stretched out to the sides.
    - Make small circles with your arms for about 10 seconds, then reverse direction.
    - Keep the movement controlled.
4. **Heel-to-Toe Walk**
    - Find a hallway or a clear space.
    - Place one foot directly in front of the other so that the heel touches the toes of the other foot.
    - Move forward slowly. Hold on to a wall for balance if you need.

These are just samples of gentle activities. If you feel any unusual pain, stop and speak with a health professional.

Moving Forward with an Active Mindset

Daily movement is about staying active in ways that fit your life and health. Whether it is walking the dog, doing a short dance, or tidying the living room, all of these can help. Moving a little bit more each day can lead to steady improvements over time.

It is not always about intense exercise routines. Many older adults find that small actions, done on a regular basis, bring noticeable benefits in how they feel. The main ideas are consistency, safety, and enjoyment. If you can find ways to make movement interesting, you are more likely to stick with it.

Chapter Summary

- **Daily Movement**: Involves regular actions like walking, housework, or simple stretches to keep the body active.
- **Body Benefits**: Helps the heart, muscles, bones, and joints function better. Can assist with weight control and overall health.
- **Mind Benefits**: Can improve mood, help with clear thinking, and reduce stress.
- **Types of Movement**: Includes walking, household tasks, chair exercises, stretching, balance work, and more.
- **Safety Tips**: Check with a doctor, wear good shoes, start slow, and pay attention to pain or dizziness.
- **Staying Motivated**: Set small goals, try fun activities, find a buddy, and track progress.
- **Overcoming Challenges**: Adjust for limited mobility, bad weather, or a busy schedule by being flexible and creative with movement choices.

By keeping these points in mind, you can make daily movement a natural part of your life. Small steps done often can offer many health gains.

CHAPTER 4: MAINTAINING A BALANCED WEIGHT

Body weight can affect many parts of health, from how we feel each day to our risk for certain problems like heart issues or strain on the joints. As people grow older, the body might not burn calories as fast as it used to. Some folks find it easier to gain extra pounds, while others lose weight too quickly due to changes in appetite. Keeping weight in a reasonable range can help improve energy levels, support the joints, and reduce the chance of problems linked to being underweight or overweight.

In this chapter, we will talk about healthy ways to manage weight over time. We will focus on practical tips for portion control, safe habits, and lifestyle factors that do not involve crash diets or extreme measures. Instead, we will look at stable methods that fit daily life and help the body feel better.

Why Does Weight Matter?

Weight is not just about appearance. It can impact how well we move, our heart's workload, and other vital aspects of health. Some people carry too much weight, which can stress knees and hips, and increase the chance of high blood pressure or diabetes. Others might be underweight, leading to a risk of weak bones or feeling tired more often. The aim is to find a balanced weight that supports overall well-being.

Understanding Metabolism in Older Age

Metabolism refers to how the body changes food and drink into energy. As we get older, our metabolism can slow down for several reasons:

1. **Less Muscle Mass**
    - Muscle tissue burns more calories than fat tissue. If we lose muscle, we burn fewer calories each day.
2. **Lifestyle Changes**
    - Some older adults may become less active, which also lowers the number of calories used.

3. **Hormonal Shifts**
    - Changes in hormone levels can affect how the body handles food and stores fat.
4. **Medical Conditions and Medications**
    - Some conditions or medicines can change appetite, digestion, or how the body uses energy.

Because of these factors, someone might gain weight even if they are eating the same amount as before. Others might not feel as hungry, leading to unplanned weight loss. Knowing this can help in making careful choices about food and activity.

Healthy Ways to Find the Right Balance

1. **Aim for Steady Progress**
    - Quick fixes are often not safe or helpful in the long run.
    - Small, steady changes in eating patterns and daily movement can keep the body healthier.
2. **Listen to Hunger Cues**
    - Some people eat out of habit, not because they are truly hungry.
    - Take time to sense whether the body really needs food. Slow down and chew carefully.
3. **Eat a Variety of Foods**
    - Different nutrients can help different processes in the body.
    - A mix of lean protein, whole grains, fruits, vegetables, and healthy fats is a good place to start.
4. **Portion Control**
    - Even nutritious foods can lead to weight gain if eaten in large amounts.
    - Use smaller plates or bowls if it helps avoid overeating.
5. **Mindful Snacking**
    - Snacks can be helpful for keeping energy up, but choose snacks like fruit, nuts, or low-fat dairy.
    - Avoid snacking while distracted (like in front of the TV), which can lead to eating more than needed.
6. **Regular Activity**
    - Pair balanced eating with some form of daily movement.
    - This helps burn extra calories and maintain muscle.

Portion Sizes Made Simple

Portion control can be confusing, especially when restaurant servings can be bigger than needed. Here are ways to manage portion sizes:

1. **Use Your Hand as a Guide**
   - A fist can represent about a cup of rice or pasta.
   - The palm of your hand (not counting fingers) can represent a serving of meat.
   - A thumb can represent a serving of cheese.
2. **Measure Food for a While**
   - Measuring cups and spoons can help you understand what a proper portion looks like.
   - After a few weeks of measuring, you might have a better sense of the right amounts.
3. **Divide Food Before Eating**
   - If you have a large package of snacks or a big meal, split it into smaller portions first.
   - Put the extra away so you are not tempted to keep eating.
4. **Eat Slowly**
   - It takes time for the brain to notice when the stomach is full.
   - Pause between bites or sips to help you recognize fullness.

Managing portion sizes does not mean starving yourself. It is about enjoying a suitable amount of food without going overboard.

Tips for Gaining Weight Safely (If Underweight)

Some older adults have the opposite problem: they might need to gain weight but are not sure how. Here are some tips:

1. **Nutrient-Dense Foods**
   - Choose items that have lots of vitamins, minerals, and healthy calories.
   - Examples include avocados, nuts, seeds, nut butters, and full-fat dairy (if tolerated).
2. **Add Small Extras**
   - Sprinkle nuts or shredded cheese onto soups or salads for extra calories.

- Use spreads like peanut butter on crackers or fruit.
3. **Frequent Meals**
    - If large meals seem too hard to finish, try having four or five smaller meals during the day.
    - Include a little protein each time.
4. **Smoothies or Shakes**
    - Blend yogurt or milk, fruit, and a spoon of peanut butter or protein powder (if allowed) for a high-calorie drink.
    - These can be easier to consume than solid foods.
5. **Address Dental Issues**
    - If chewing is hard, softer foods like mashed potatoes, cooked vegetables, or soups can help.
    - Talk to a dentist if teeth or dentures cause problems.

If someone is underweight due to a health condition or loss of appetite, seeking help from a medical professional can provide a personalized approach.

Dealing with Weight Gain or Obesity

For those who have too much extra weight, simple steps can help:

1. **Focus on Gradual Changes**
    - Avoid drastic diets that promise quick results.
    - Try cutting back on sugary drinks or desserts one step at a time.
2. **Make Simple Swaps**
    - Use spices or herbs instead of butter or cream sauces for flavor.
    - Choose water or unsweetened tea instead of soda.
3. **Watch Out for Liquid Calories**
    - Drinks like sweet tea, fruit juice, or flavored coffee can add lots of sugar without filling you up.
    - Stick with low-calorie or no-calorie beverages.
4. **Include Protein in Meals**
    - Protein can help you feel full longer.
    - Lean meats, fish, beans, and eggs are good choices.
5. **Plan for Indulgences**
    - It is okay to enjoy a treat now and then.
    - Keep track of how often and how much you have so it does not become an everyday habit.
6. **Stay Active**

- Combine lower-calorie eating with some daily movement to help with weight loss or prevent more gain.
- Look for enjoyable activities like walks or gentle dancing.

Staying motivated might be easier if you have a friend or relative who supports your goals. Some also find help through community programs that focus on safe, slow weight loss for older adults.

Emotional Factors Around Weight

Weight is sometimes tied to feelings. People might eat to handle stress or sadness. Older adults might also face changes in life that affect mood, leading to problems like overeating or not eating enough. Paying attention to emotional signals can make a difference:

1. **Identify Emotional Eating**
    - Notice if you are eating because you are bored, lonely, or upset instead of actually hungry.
    - Try to handle feelings in other ways, like calling a friend or going for a walk.
2. **Seek Support**
    - Talking with a counselor or a support group can help if emotions are affecting your eating habits.
    - Friends or family members can offer a listening ear or help with healthy meal ideas.
3. **Create Enjoyable Routines**
    - If you feel lonely at mealtime, try sharing meals with someone or chatting on the phone.
    - Small social connections can reduce emotional eating.

Sometimes, deeper problems like grief or depression can change how a person eats. If that is the case, it might be wise to get professional help to address the main cause.

Checking Progress Without Stress

Weighing yourself can help track changes, but it should be done in a healthy way:

1. **Weigh Yourself Weekly**
   - Weighing every day can cause stress due to natural daily swings in weight.
   - Once a week, at the same time of day, is enough to see a trend.
2. **Look at Long-Term Patterns**
   - If your weight goes up or down by a small amount once in a while, it might not matter.
   - Keep an eye on shifts over several weeks or months to see a real pattern.
3. **Note How Clothes Fit**
   - Sometimes the scale number does not tell the full story.
   - If your clothes feel tighter or looser, that might indicate a body change.
4. **Other Health Measures**
   - Blood sugar levels, blood pressure, and cholesterol numbers can also show progress.
   - Feeling more energetic or sleeping better can be another sign that you are on the right track.

Try not to become fixated on the scale. Weight is only one sign of overall health.

The Role of Balanced Meals and Snacks

Balanced meals can help keep weight in a normal range. Each meal should ideally have:

- **Protein** (like chicken, fish, eggs, beans)
- **Healthy Carbs** (like whole grains, fruits, or vegetables)
- **A Little Fat** (like a small amount of nuts, avocado, or olive oil)

Snacks can fit in if they are chosen wisely. For instance, an apple with peanut butter provides carbs, protein, and fat. A snack of chips might be less filling, leading you to eat more later. Balancing meals in a regular pattern also stops big hunger swings that could make you overeat.

Putting Activity and Weight Management Together

Earlier, we covered how daily movement can support the body. When mixed with wiser eating, it can help balance weight:

1. **Burn More Calories**
    - Even short walks or simple tasks help burn some extra energy.
    - The more you move, the more you offset the calories you eat.
2. **Build Muscle**
    - Exercises that work the muscles can raise metabolism slightly, helping you burn more calories at rest.
    - Muscle also supports better balance and daily function.
3. **Improved Mood**
    - Activity can help reduce stress, which might lower emotional eating.
    - Feeling good often leads to better choices around food.
4. **Better Sleep**
    - Good rest can help control hormones that affect hunger and appetite.
    - Activity during the day can lead to better sleep at night.

It is often easier to manage weight when you address both food intake and physical activity. Small steps in each area can add up.

Ideas for Ongoing Success

1. **Set Realistic Goals**
    - Maybe aim to lose 1 or 2 pounds a month if you need to lose weight, or gain a bit each month if you need to gain.
    - Sudden changes can stress the body.
2. **Track What You Eat**
    - Some people find it helpful to jot down meals in a food diary.
    - This can make you more aware of snacking or patterns that lead to overeating.
3. **Stay Hydrated**
    - Thirst can sometimes feel like hunger.
    - Drinking water regularly helps keep your body balanced.
4. **Plan Meals Ahead**

- If you know what you are going to eat, you are less likely to pick something unhealthy at the last minute.
- Planning helps you manage portions and ensure variety.
5. **Seek Medical Advice**
    - If you have diabetes, heart issues, or other medical conditions, talk to your doctor about weight targets.
    - A dietitian or nutritionist can give specialized plans.

Avoiding Extreme Diets

Fad diets that cut out entire food groups or promise very fast results can cause harm. They can lead to missing nutrients, low energy, or other issues. Some extreme diets may also cause quick weight loss followed by weight regain. Instead, focus on balance and a slow, steady approach. This is often more gentle on the body and can be sustained over time.

Common Pitfalls

1. **Skipping Meals**
    - This can cause big hunger swings and lead to overeating later.
    - Having balanced meals at regular times can prevent that.
2. **Relying on Sweets for Quick Energy**
    - Sugary snacks might boost energy briefly, then cause a crash.
    - Consider whole grain crackers, fruit, or nuts for a steadier source of energy.
3. **Eating Too Few Calories**
    - If you severely cut calories, you could feel weak or dizzy.
    - You also risk losing muscle if you do not eat enough protein.
4. **Ignoring Liquid Intake**
    - Not drinking enough water can slow metabolism and make it harder to lose weight (if that is the goal).
    - Dehydration can also make you feel sluggish.
5. **Unrealistic Expectations**
    - Aiming to drop several pounds each week is not safe for most older adults.
    - Focus on slow changes and overall wellness.

Knowing When to Ask for Professional Help

Some people find it hard to manage weight on their own. It might be helpful to ask a doctor or dietitian for guidance if:

- You have a sudden change in weight without a clear reason.
- You feel tired or weak often.
- You have a health condition (like diabetes or kidney issues) that needs a specific meal plan.
- You are unsure if you should lose or gain weight.

A professional can check if there are medical causes behind weight changes and suggest solutions tailored to your needs.

Chapter Summary

- **Metabolism and Aging**: As we age, metabolism can slow down, and muscle mass may decrease. This affects how we gain or lose weight.
- **Healthy Balance**: Aim for a reasonable weight that supports energy and joint health.
- **Practical Tips**:
    - For **overweight**: Use portion control, watch sugary drinks, stay active, and make gradual diet changes.
    - For **underweight**: Choose nutrient-dense foods, eat smaller but more frequent meals, and address any chewing problems.
- **Mindful Eating**: Listen to hunger cues and be aware of emotional eating.
- **Activity and Weight**: Daily movement works with healthy eating to manage weight.
- **Professional Support**: Doctors and dietitians can guide you if you have medical conditions or need more help.

Maintaining a balanced weight is not about strict rules. It is about understanding your body's needs, making steady improvements, and looking for help when needed. With practical steps, you can find a weight range that supports feeling better in day-to-day life.

CHAPTER 5: HEART HEALTH AND BLOOD PRESSURE TIPS

The heart is like the engine of our bodies. It pumps blood to all our organs and tissues, bringing oxygen and nutrients so we can function. As people get older, the heart and blood vessels can face new challenges. Some folks may develop high blood pressure or have heart conditions that need extra attention. Learning about heart health can help prevent problems or keep them from getting worse.

In this chapter, we will look at common issues that affect the heart, with a special focus on blood pressure. We will talk about what can make blood pressure rise, why it matters, and what you can do about it. We will also cover tips that support overall heart health, such as choosing the right types of foods, staying active, and managing stress in ways that do not repeat advice from earlier chapters.

Why Heart Health Matters

The heart is always working. It pumps blood day and night without rest. Because it works nonstop, we must take care of it. When the heart has problems, a person may feel tired or weak. In serious cases, heart problems can lead to sudden medical emergencies like heart attacks. However, many risks can be lowered by paying attention to what we eat, how much we move, and other factors in daily life.

Being aware of heart health is important at any age, but especially as we get older. The blood vessels, which carry blood to every part of the body, can become stiffer or narrower over time. That can raise blood pressure or create blockages that strain the heart. Good lifestyle habits can help keep things in balance.

Understanding Blood Pressure

Blood pressure measures the force of blood pushing against the walls of your blood vessels. It is measured using two numbers:

- **Systolic** (the top number): The pressure when the heart beats and pushes blood out.
- **Diastolic** (the bottom number): The pressure when the heart rests between beats.

For example, a reading might be 120/80 mmHg (said as "120 over 80"). This is often considered a normal range for many adults. If the top number (systolic) is 130 or higher, or the bottom number (diastolic) is 80 or higher, that can mean you have high blood pressure (also called hypertension). Doctors might watch these numbers closely to decide if you need changes in your habits or medication.

Why High Blood Pressure Can Be a Problem

High blood pressure often has no clear signs at first. People sometimes call it a "silent" issue because you might not feel anything unusual until the problem becomes serious. Over time, the strain of high blood pressure can damage blood vessels and organs like the kidneys or eyes. It can also raise the chances of heart attacks or strokes.

For older adults, changes in blood vessels or hormones can make high blood pressure more likely. Some people also find that certain medicines affect blood pressure. If left untreated, high blood pressure can quietly hurt the heart and other systems. That is why getting your blood pressure checked regularly is key.

Common Causes of High Blood Pressure

1. **Unhealthy Eating Habits**
    - Diets with too much salt or unhealthy fats can increase the risk of high blood pressure.
    - Too many sugary drinks or refined carbohydrates might also play a role.
2. **Lack of Movement**
    - When we do not move often, the heart and blood vessels can become weaker and less flexible.
    - This may contribute to higher blood pressure over time.
3. **Excess Weight**

- Carrying extra pounds can put more stress on the heart and circulation.
- This can raise blood pressure and strain the body.
4. **Family History**
    - High blood pressure can run in families.
    - Even if there is a genetic tendency, healthy habits can lower the risk.
5. **Older Age**
    - Arteries can get stiffer or narrower as we age, leading to higher pressure.
    - This does not mean everyone will have high blood pressure, but it becomes more common.
6. **Other Health Conditions**
    - Conditions like kidney disease or diabetes can affect blood pressure.
    - Some medications can also cause changes in pressure.

Understanding these causes can help us make choices that lower risks. While we cannot change our age or genes, we can work on our habits and see a doctor if health issues arise.

Practical Tips for Healthier Blood Pressure

Below are methods to help keep blood pressure in a safe range. We will try not to overlap with previous chapters too much, but some basic themes cannot be avoided. These tips highlight areas unique to blood pressure control:

1. **Watch Your Sodium (Salt) Intake**
    - Sodium can be found in table salt and in many packaged foods.
    - Limit the use of canned soups or sauces that list sodium in large amounts on the label.
    - Use fresh or dried herbs instead of salt for flavor. For example, season chicken with garlic powder and a bit of black pepper instead of extra salt.
2. **Focus on Heart-Helpful Foods**
    - Increase foods that have potassium, such as bananas, sweet potatoes, or spinach. Potassium can help balance sodium levels in the body.

- Choose meals that include lean proteins, whole grains, and plenty of fruits and vegetables.
- Look for "low sodium" or "no salt added" labels on items like tomato sauce or beans.

3. **Stay Hydrated**
    - Drinking enough water helps the body get rid of extra sodium.
    - Try to sip water throughout the day rather than chugging large amounts at once.
4. **Mindful Beverage Choices**
    - Certain drinks can affect blood pressure. Caffeine (in coffee or tea) might raise it for a short time.
    - Alcohol can raise blood pressure if taken in large amounts, so limit it according to your doctor's advice.
5. **Consider Heart-Friendly Herbs or Flavors**
    - Many herbs and spices can add taste without raising blood pressure.
    - Examples: basil, oregano, thyme, onion powder, lemon juice, or vinegar.
6. **Adequate Sleep**
    - Sleep problems can raise stress hormones, which might lead to higher blood pressure over time.
    - Aim for a sleep routine that feels restful.
7. **Regular Blood Pressure Checks**
    - Visit your doctor or pharmacy to check blood pressure regularly.
    - If you have a home monitor, follow instructions carefully to get accurate readings.
    - Keep a record of readings to see patterns or changes.

Other Heart-Healthy Tips Beyond Blood Pressure

Even if your blood pressure is normal, there are more ways to keep your heart strong:

1. **Know Your Cholesterol Levels**
    - Cholesterol is a fat-like substance in the blood. High levels can lead to clogs in arteries.
    - A test can show your total cholesterol, including "good" (HDL) and "bad" (LDL) cholesterol.

- Eating fewer saturated and trans fats can help manage cholesterol. Foods like fatty cuts of meat or baked goods with hydrogenated oils can raise "bad" cholesterol.
2. **Stay Active in Ways That Help the Heart**
    - Activities like walking, gentle biking, or water exercises can strengthen the heart without too much strain.
    - Gradually increase the time you spend on these movements, aiming for safe progress.
3. **Watch Out for Triggers**
    - Stressful situations might affect the heart. Recognizing what causes stress can help you find ways to calm down.
    - Some easy calming actions can include slow, deep breathing or listening to soothing music.
4. **Limit Solid Fats and Sugar**
    - Foods like butter, lard, and sweets can add unwanted calories and raise cholesterol or blood sugar.
    - Replace them with unsaturated fats found in avocados or nuts if you want some flavor and healthy fats.
5. **Be Careful with Over-the-Counter Medicines**
    - Some cold or pain medications can raise blood pressure or strain the heart.
    - Check labels or talk with a pharmacist about safe options for you.

Working with Your Healthcare Provider

Doctors can be partners in protecting your heart. Here is how you can team up with them:

1. **Regular Appointments**
    - Get check-ups even if you feel fine. Early detection of problems can prevent serious issues.
    - Ask about heart tests like ECG (electrocardiogram) or blood tests if recommended.
2. **Medication Management**
    - If you are given medicine for blood pressure or any heart condition, follow the instructions closely.
    - Let the doctor know if you have side effects like dizziness or swelling.

- Never stop a medication suddenly without checking with a healthcare professional.
3. **Ask Questions**
    - If the doctor suggests changes in your diet or daily habits, ask for details.
    - Write down advice so you can remember it later.
4. **Report Symptoms**
    - Pain in the chest, heavy feeling in the arms, or feeling faint can all be warning signs.
    - Seek help right away if you experience something alarming.

Signs of Heart-Related Trouble

Being aware of warning signs can help you catch issues early or act fast in emergencies:

1. **Chest Discomfort**
    - Pain, pressure, or squeezing in the chest that might spread to the arms or jaw.
    - Sometimes it might feel like indigestion or heartburn.
2. **Shortness of Breath**
    - Feeling like you cannot catch your breath even when you are not doing much.
    - This could be a sign that the heart or lungs are working too hard.
3. **Feeling Lightheaded or Dizzy**
    - Sudden dizziness or faintness might mean blood flow to the brain is not enough.
    - It can also happen when blood pressure drops too low or spikes too high.
4. **Swelling in the Legs or Ankles**
    - The heart might not be pumping well, causing fluid buildup in the lower body.
5. **Unusual Fatigue**
    - Feeling extra tired after normal tasks could mean the heart is not supplying enough oxygen.

If you notice any of these signs, especially if they come on suddenly, consider seeking medical help right away.

Simple Ways to Protect the Heart Each Day

You do not need big changes overnight. Try adding small steps that can help protect your heart:

1. **Plan Heart-Healthy Meals**
   - When making a grocery list, include fruits, vegetables, and lean proteins.
   - Use herbs and spices instead of salt when cooking.
2. **Set a Reminder for Movement**
   - Even if you only have five minutes, a brief walk or light stretching can help circulation.
   - Try to stand up at least once an hour if you are sitting for long periods.
3. **Check Labels for Sodium**
   - Many packaged foods have more sodium than we realize.
   - Compare brands and pick ones with lower sodium when possible.
4. **Practice Calm Breathing**
   - Sit comfortably, inhale slowly through the nose, then exhale gently through the mouth.
   - Do this a few times to help steady the mind and reduce tension.
5. **Stay Connected**
   - Chat with friends or family. Positive relationships can help reduce stress.
   - Consider joining a social club or activity group if you feel isolated.
6. **Keep Track of Appointments**
   - Use a calendar or notebook to remember doctor visits, medication refills, or lab tests.
   - Being organized helps prevent missed check-ups.

Different Approaches to Stress Management

Stress can make the heart work harder. While we have mentioned some general tips in previous chapters, here are a few fresh ideas:

1. **Warm Bath Soak**
   - A warm bath can relax tense muscles and calm the mind.
   - Make sure the water is not too hot, especially if you have blood pressure concerns.

- Soak for a short period, like 10 to 15 minutes.
2. **Gentle Hobbies for Calmness**
    - Activities like coloring in a simple coloring book, sorting through family photos, or rearranging small items on a shelf can be soothing.
    - These tasks focus the mind on something pleasant, which helps dial down stress.
3. **Stay in Touch with Nature**
    - A few minutes of fresh air, even on a balcony or porch, can help clear your head.
    - Looking at plants or a garden can also have a calming effect.
4. **Short Mental Breaks**
    - If you feel overwhelmed, close your eyes and picture a place that makes you feel at ease, such as a quiet beach or a peaceful meadow.
    - This mini mental vacation can lower stress quickly.
5. **Stretching Before Bed**
    - Doing a couple of slow stretches can release tension from the day.
    - This may help you sleep more soundly, which in turn supports heart health.

Managing Blood Pressure Medications

Some people may need medication to control blood pressure. Here are pointers if that is part of your plan:

1. **Follow the Schedule**
    - Take medicine at the same time each day if possible.
    - Use a pill organizer or a timer on your phone to avoid missing doses.
2. **Know Possible Side Effects**
    - Some medications can cause dry cough, dizziness, or other effects.
    - Keep track of how you feel and tell your doctor if something is not right.
3. **Do Not Skip Doses**
    - Stopping blood pressure medication suddenly can lead to a big spike in pressure.
    - Always check with the doctor if you think a change is needed.

4. **Lifestyle Changes Still Matter**
   - Medication helps, but it does not replace healthy eating, movement, or stress control.
   - Combining medication with good habits often leads to better results.

Avoiding Tobacco in Any Form

Smoking or using other tobacco products can harm the heart. It can:

- Narrow blood vessels, raising blood pressure
- Lower oxygen levels in the blood
- Make it easier for clots to form, which can lead to heart attacks or strokes

If you smoke, talk with a healthcare professional about programs or medication that can help you stop. Quitting tobacco can bring improvements in heart health at any age. Even if you have been a smoker for years, stopping can lower the risk of further damage to your heart and lungs.

How to Measure Your Blood Pressure at Home

If your doctor suggests checking blood pressure at home, the right method can lead to more accurate results:

1. **Pick a Good Machine**
   - Many drugstores sell automatic blood pressure cuffs for the upper arm.
   - Choose one labeled "clinically validated."
2. **Follow Instructions**
   - Sit quietly for a few minutes before measuring.
   - Support your arm on a flat surface so the cuff is at heart level.
3. **Record Readings**
   - Write down the date, time, and your result.
   - If the readings are often high or too low, let your doctor know.
4. **Take Multiple Readings**
   - Two or three measurements a minute apart can show a more reliable number.

    - Average them if they differ by a lot.

Early Warning: Low Blood Pressure

While high blood pressure is more common, low blood pressure can also be dangerous for some individuals. Low blood pressure might cause:

- Dizziness
- Weakness
- Fainting
- Blurry vision

If you notice these problems, your doctor can help figure out the cause. Sometimes, certain medications for high blood pressure or heart issues can make pressure drop too low, especially if you stand up too quickly. In other cases, dehydration or other problems may be at fault.

Keeping a Heart-Healthy Mindset

Building habits that protect the heart is a process, but it can become part of normal life:

- **Set small goals.** For example, aim to reduce sodium in one meal each day or take a short walk after lunch.
- **Stay informed.** Read reliable sources about heart health, ask your doctor questions, and keep up with the latest recommendations for older adults.
- **Check in with yourself.** Notice if stress, fatigue, or other factors are creeping in. Adjust your routine as needed to stay balanced.

Over time, these steps become a part of daily life. The heart will be better prepared to handle challenges if it is well cared for.

CHAPTER 6: CARING FOR BONES AND JOINTS

Bones and joints form the framework that holds us upright and allows movement. Over the years, they can face wear and tear. This might lead to conditions like osteoporosis, which makes bones weaker, or arthritis, which can cause joint pain and stiffness. Learning how to care for bones and joints can improve comfort and mobility as we age.

In this chapter, we will look at why bones become more fragile, how joints can get stiff or painful, and simple steps to support bone and joint health. We will include details about posture, safe activities, and how to handle common concerns without repeating what we have shared in earlier chapters.

The Basics of Bones

1. **Structure**
   - Bones are living tissues that rebuild themselves.
   - Inside them is bone marrow, which makes blood cells and stores minerals like calcium.
2. **Bone Density**
   - In childhood and early adulthood, the body builds bone mass.
   - After a certain point, we might lose bone faster than we make it if we do not watch our diet, exercise, and other factors.
3. **Osteoporosis**
   - A condition where bones become thinner and break more easily.
   - Common in older adults, especially women after certain hormonal changes.
   - It does not happen to everyone, but many people have some level of bone loss.
4. **Calcium and Vitamin D**
   - Calcium strengthens bones, and vitamin D helps the body take in calcium.
   - Getting enough of these nutrients can slow bone loss.
   - Spending a small amount of time in sunlight helps the body produce vitamin D, but be mindful of sun exposure limits to protect skin.

The Basics of Joints

1. **How Joints Work**
   - Joints are where two bones come together.
   - Many joints have cartilage, a smooth material that helps bones glide without rubbing directly.
2. **Types of Joints**
   - Knees, hips, shoulders, and elbows are examples of joints that move in different ways.
   - Some joints, like those in the skull, are fixed and do not move.
3. **Arthritis**
   - A common condition that causes pain, swelling, or stiffness in joints.
   - There are various forms of arthritis, but osteoarthritis is often linked to age-related wear on cartilage.
   - Another form, rheumatoid arthritis, involves the immune system and can harm joint tissues.
4. **Cartilage and Cushioning**
   - Cartilage can wear down over time, leading to bones rubbing against each other, which causes pain.
   - In some joints, fluid (called synovial fluid) adds lubrication to prevent friction.

Signs Your Bones or Joints Need Attention

1. **Joint Pain or Swelling**
   - Pain in a joint that lasts more than a few days, especially with swelling or redness, should be checked.
2. **Reduced Range of Motion**
   - If you cannot bend or straighten a joint as much as before, it might be due to stiffness or a problem in the joint.
3. **Bone Fractures After Minor Falls**
   - Breaking a bone from a minor slip can be a warning sign of weak bones.
4. **Stooped Posture**
   - A rounded back or a stooped posture might mean the spine's bones are weaker or compressed.

If you notice these issues, a doctor might suggest scans (like a bone density test) or other exams to diagnose the problem.

Nutrients That Support Bone and Joint Health

While we spoke about nutrition in an earlier chapter, here we will focus on specific nutrients for bones and joints:

1. **Calcium**
    - Helps keep bones firm and strong.
    - Found in dairy products, fortified plant milks, and leafy green vegetables.
    - Recommended intake varies with age, so check with a doctor for personal needs.
2. **Vitamin D**
    - Aids the body in taking in calcium.
    - Found in fatty fish, egg yolks, and fortified foods.
    - The body also makes vitamin D from limited sun exposure.
3. **Protein**
    - Essential for building bone tissue and muscle that supports joints.
    - Good sources include lean meats, beans, lentils, and dairy.
    - Spreading out protein intake across meals can help the body use it more effectively.
4. **Omega-3 Fatty Acids**
    - These healthy fats can help reduce inflammation in joints.
    - Found in oily fish like salmon or sardines, as well as in flaxseeds or walnuts.
5. **Antioxidants**
    - Vitamins C and E can help protect joint tissues from damage.
    - Colorful fruits and vegetables often provide these.

A balanced approach that includes these nutrients can give bones and joints the support they need. If a person struggles to get enough from food, a doctor might suggest supplements.

Lifestyle Habits for Bone and Joint Support

1. **Stay Active (in a Safe Way)**
    - Movement helps bones and joints stay strong and flexible.
    - Weight-bearing exercises like walking or simple stair climbing can boost bone density.

- Low-impact activities (such as water exercises) help joints move without too much stress.
2. **Keep a Healthy Posture**
    - Sitting or standing in a slumped position can strain the spine.
    - Practice sitting upright with shoulders back and chin level.
    - When bending or lifting items, use your legs instead of your back to lower stress on the spine.
3. **Maintain a Suitable Weight**
    - Extra pounds can strain knees, hips, and ankles, making joint problems worse.
    - On the other hand, being too thin can harm bone strength.
    - Aim for a weight range that your doctor thinks is right for your build and health status.
4. **Avoid Smoking**
    - Smoking can reduce bone mass and make osteoporosis more likely.
    - It may also harm circulation, which can affect joint tissues.
5. **Watch Alcohol Use**
    - Heavy drinking can interfere with how bones rebuild themselves and might lead to weaker bones.
    - Alcohol can also raise the risk of falls and fractures.

Specific Exercises for Bones and Joints

Here are exercises that focus on strengthening or preserving bone and joint health. (We will avoid repeating the daily movement details from Chapter 3 as much as possible and focus on new specifics.)

1. **Weight-Bearing Walks**
    - Walking is a gentle way to apply pressure on bones, encouraging them to stay strong.
    - Consider adding small hills or gentle slopes if your doctor says it is safe. This slight increase in effort can benefit hips and legs.
2. **Seated Knee Extensions for Joint Stability**
    - Sit in a sturdy chair, straighten one leg in front of you, hold for a moment, then lower it.
    - This can help strengthen the muscles around the knees.
    - Do it slowly to avoid jerking the joint.

3. **Heel Raises for Ankle Support**
    - Stand behind a chair for balance. Rise up onto your toes, then lower your heels back down.
    - This supports calf muscles and helps keep ankles stable.
4. **Gentle Resistance Bands**
    - Use a band to do slow bicep curls or shoulder presses.
    - This helps build muscle that protects bones and keeps joints moving well.
5. **Hip Flexor Stretches**
    - Kneel on one knee (use padding if needed), with the other foot flat on the ground in front.
    - Slowly shift weight forward to feel a stretch in the hip. This can ease stiffness in the hip joint.

Always speak to a healthcare provider before starting new exercises if you have existing bone or joint conditions. Proper form is crucial to avoid injury.

Handling Joint Discomfort

Mild joint discomfort might happen from time to time. Here are some methods that can offer relief without duplicating earlier tips:

1. **Warm Compresses**
    - Applying a warm towel or a heating pad can loosen tight muscles around the joint.
    - Use warmth for about 15 minutes at a time.
2. **Cool Packs**
    - If swelling is present, placing a cool pack can reduce inflammation.
    - Wrap ice or frozen veggies in a thin cloth rather than placing them directly on the skin.
3. **Topical Creams**
    - Some over-the-counter creams have ingredients like menthol or capsaicin, which can numb minor joint pain.
    - Test a small spot first to check for irritation.
4. **Gentle Massage**
    - Lightly rubbing around the joint can increase blood flow.
    - Avoid pressing directly on the joint if it is very tender.
5. **Alternate Rest and Movement**

- Too much rest can make joints stiffer, while too much activity might increase pain.
- Finding a balance can improve how the joint feels overall.

If pain lasts or worsens, it is best to talk to a doctor for further guidance.

A Note on Supplements for Bones and Joints

Many products claim to support bone and joint health. Some popular ones include calcium pills, vitamin D tablets, and substances like glucosamine or chondroitin for joint comfort. Before trying any new supplement:

- **Speak to a Healthcare Professional**: They can tell you if the supplement is safe based on your medical history.
- **Check Dosages**: Too much of certain vitamins, like vitamin D, can be harmful.
- **Watch Out for Drug Interactions**: Some supplements might interfere with prescriptions.

Relying too heavily on supplements without changing habits (like diet or exercise) is not recommended. A balanced approach usually works best.

Preventing Falls to Protect Bones

A fall can break bones, especially if they are already weakened. Lower the risk of falls with these ideas:

1. **Keep Floors Clear**
   - Remove loose rugs or secure them with non-slip backing.
   - Keep walkways free of cords or clutter.
2. **Good Lighting**
   - Put bright bulbs in areas like stairwells or hallways.
   - Use nightlights in the bathroom and bedroom so you can see if you get up at night.
3. **Safe Footwear**
   - Wear shoes with non-slip soles.
   - Avoid high heels or loose slippers that can increase the chance of tripping.

4. **Handrails and Support**
    - Install grab bars in the bathroom if needed.
    - Use a stable cane or walker if balance is an issue.
5. **Eye Check-Ups**
    - Clear vision helps you notice hazards.
    - Update your eyeglasses if your prescription changes.

Staying aware of your surroundings is a simple way to protect bones by avoiding harmful accidents.

Dealing with Osteoporosis

If you have osteoporosis or are at high risk, here are key points:

1. **Bone Density Tests**
    - A DEXA scan measures how thick or thin your bones are.
    - Your doctor might order one if you have risk factors.
2. **Medications for Bone Health**
    - Some drugs slow bone loss or help build new bone.
    - Common examples include bisphosphonates or hormone-related treatments.
    - Discuss benefits and side effects with your doctor.
3. **Weight-Bearing Exercise**
    - Even short walks or gentle lifting of small weights can stimulate bone growth.
    - Swimming is good for joints, but it does not stress bones as much as activities on land.
4. **Lifestyle Checks**
    - Smoking and heavy alcohol use can worsen bone density.
    - Address these factors if they apply to you.
5. **Protect Yourself**
    - If bones break easily, be extra cautious about fall risks.
    - Wear supportive shoes and keep your home free of tripping hazards.

Osteoporosis does not have to mean giving up on favorite activities. With the right care, many people continue to enjoy life while managing bone health carefully.

Coping with Arthritis

Arthritis can be managed in various ways:

1. **Medications**
   - Over-the-counter pain relievers might help mild arthritis.
   - Stronger prescriptions or anti-inflammatory drugs might be needed in some cases.
   - A doctor can suggest medication based on the type of arthritis.
2. **Physical Therapy**
   - A physical therapist can show safe exercises that keep joints flexible.
   - They might also use techniques like ultrasound or massage to reduce pain.
3. **Tools for Easier Living**
   - Devices like jar openers or button hooks can lessen strain on painful joints.
   - A cane, walker, or special braces might provide extra support.
4. **Activity Choices**
   - Low-impact activities, such as swimming or light cycling, can keep joints moving without too much stress.
   - Avoid sudden, jerky actions that can irritate the joints.
5. **Heat and Cold Therapy**
   - Some people find relief by alternating warm and cool packs.
   - Ask a healthcare professional about the best schedule for applying them.

Arthritis varies from person to person, so it may take time to find the right methods that work best for you.

Strengthening Supporting Muscles

Strong muscles around a joint can help stabilize it and lower pain. Some suggestions:

1. **Focus on Core Muscles**
   - The muscles in the abdomen and lower back help support the spine and hips.

- Simple exercises like slow abdominal tightening or safe plank variations can build this area.
2. **Strengthen Thigh Muscles**
   - Squats or sitting-to-standing motions can help if done with good form.
   - Strong thighs reduce stress on the knees.
3. **Work on Shoulders and Upper Back**
   - Light resistance band exercises that focus on the shoulder blades can improve posture.
   - This helps reduce neck and shoulder strain.
4. **Balance Muscle Groups**
   - Train both the front and back parts of the body. For instance, strengthen both chest and upper back muscles.
   - Balanced muscles keep joints aligned.

A physical therapist or trainer experienced with older adults can create a routine that targets supporting muscles without risking injury.

When to Seek Professional Help

Sometimes bone or joint pain needs more than home care:

1. **Severe or Lasting Pain**
   - If pain does not improve with rest, gentle movement, or basic remedies, it might need special attention.
2. **Sudden Swelling or Redness**
   - This could mean inflammation or infection in the joint.
   - Seek medical advice if it appears suddenly.
3. **Cracking or Popping Sensations**
   - Occasional crackles might be normal, but if they come with pain, see a doctor.
4. **Trouble Doing Everyday Tasks**
   - If getting dressed, climbing stairs, or cooking becomes too hard due to bone or joint issues, professional help can guide you.
5. **Frequent Falls**
   - More than one or two falls in a short period might signal balance or bone health problems.

Doctors, physical therapists, or orthopedic specialists can diagnose the root cause and offer targeted treatments.

CHAPTER 7: SUPPORTING BRAIN HEALTH AND MEMORY

Our brains help us think, remember, and handle daily tasks. As we get older, the brain can change in ways that affect memory, attention, and other abilities. Some folks may notice that they misplace items more often or have trouble recalling names. Others might feel like it takes longer to learn something new. These changes can be normal, but there are steps we can take to support the brain and keep it as strong as possible.

In this chapter, we will look at the reasons why some memory problems happen with age, discuss healthy habits that can help the brain, and offer ideas for making day-to-day tasks easier. We will also look at ways to keep the mind engaged and focused, without repeating advice from earlier chapters on stress or physical movement. By exploring fresh approaches, you can find new tips that may fit your needs.

How the Brain Changes with Age

1. **Slower Processing Speed**
    - As we grow older, signals in the brain might move more slowly.
    - This can make it seem like you need extra time to learn new skills or switch between tasks.
2. **Short-Term Memory Gaps**
    - Some older adults find it harder to recall new information, such as a phone number or a recent conversation.
    - Often, long-term memories (like childhood events) stay more stable, while short-term recall might fade faster.
3. **Reduced Blood Flow**
    - The blood vessels in the brain can become less flexible, possibly affecting oxygen and nutrient delivery.
    - This may contribute to feeling mentally tired during certain tasks.
4. **Changes in Brain Cells**
    - Over time, certain parts of the brain can shrink slightly. The brain may not repair cells as quickly as in youth.
    - But many cells continue working well, and the brain can form new connections, known as "neuroplasticity," even in later years.

Not everyone faces the same changes at the same pace. Genetics, environment, and daily habits all play a role in how the brain ages.

Common Memory Concerns

1. **Forgetting Names and Faces**
   - Many older adults find themselves saying, "I know that person, but I can't recall the name."
   - This might happen simply because the brain needs more time to link details.
2. **Misplacing Items**
   - Losing keys, glasses, or the remote can happen at any age, but it may feel more common later on.
   - Often, this is related to not paying full attention when putting things down.
3. **Word-Finding Difficulties**
   - You might pause mid-sentence searching for the right word.
   - This can be normal, though it may feel frustrating.
4. **Difficulty Focusing**
   - Following a lengthy discussion or staying on task might seem harder.
   - Distractions can pull attention away more easily.

Minor lapses are a typical part of aging. However, if memory problems severely disrupt daily life, such as forgetting common words very often or becoming confused in familiar places, it might be wise to seek medical advice.

Ways to Support Brain Health

The brain benefits from a range of positive habits. While some general wellness tips have been mentioned in other chapters, here are new details specific to the mind:

1. **Challenge the Mind with Variety**
   - Try new brain tasks that you have not done before. For example, if you usually do word puzzles, consider trying a simple language-learning app or a new style of brainteaser.

- Switching between different types of mental tasks can help the brain form new connections.
2. **Stay Curious**
	- Pick up short articles or watch documentaries on topics you do not know much about.
	- Jot down interesting facts to share with a friend. This process helps you engage with new information and remember it more clearly.
3. **Break Learning into Steps**
	- If you want to learn something new—like a simple computer skill—divide it into small stages.
	- Focus on one stage at a time, rather than trying to absorb everything all at once.
4. **Practice Recall**
	- After reading something, pause and try to restate the key points in your own words.
	- This can strengthen the memory of what you just learned.
5. **Use Multiple Senses**
	- If possible, pair what you want to remember with a visual or a sound. For instance, if you want to remember a new recipe, read the steps out loud and look at pictures of the ingredients.
	- The more senses involved, the stronger the memory link might be.
6. **Limit Interruptions**
	- If focusing is hard, create a quiet space. Turn off the TV or put your phone away for a while.
	- Even short breaks in attention can make it tougher to store information in memory.

Keeping the Brain Active in Everyday Life

Supporting brain health does not require fancy classes or expensive gadgets. Small, daily actions can help:

1. **Mental Notes**
	- Each morning, think about a simple goal for the day, like making a call or sorting out a drawer. Remember that goal and try to stick with it.
	- This small act trains the mind to set and recall tasks.

2. **Reading with Purpose**
   - When reading a newspaper or a magazine, pick one article and focus on key details.
   - Test yourself afterward by seeing how much you can restate without looking back.
3. **Create an Organized Environment**
   - Keep frequently used items (like keys) in the same place to lower mental strain and free your brain for more complex tasks.
   - Label boxes or shelves if you have trouble remembering where things go.
4. **Use Simple Tools**
   - Calendars or planners can help track appointments and tasks.
   - Sticky notes on the bathroom mirror or kitchen cabinet can remind you of daily tasks (like taking vitamins).
5. **Engage in Meaningful Social Chats**
   - Talking with someone about a shared interest can stimulate the brain.
   - Ask them questions that make you think, and share your own thoughts in return.

Handling Stress for Better Thinking

While we have discussed stress in previous chapters, here are fresh tips that focus on how stress affects thinking:

1. **Focus on One Task**
   - Multi-tasking can overload the brain, especially when stress is present.
   - Finish one thing before moving to the next whenever you can.
2. **Brief Mind Breaks**
   - In addition to calm breathing, try closing your eyes and counting slowly to 10.
   - Visualize a simple shape in your mind (like a square), and picture each side as you count.
3. **Pair Tasks with Something Pleasant**
   - If you have a routine chore that causes mild stress, like folding laundry, play gentle background music.

- Keep the music low enough so you can still focus, but let it give a pleasant mood to the task.
4. **Stick to a Reasonable Schedule**
    - Spreading out big tasks can help lower mental clutter.
    - Avoid scheduling back-to-back activities if you feel rushed.

When stress is high, thinking and remembering can get tougher. Finding ways to ease stress can, in turn, help with clearer thought and better recall.

The Role of Sleep in Brain Health

Sleep gives the brain time to sort and store information. Here are some ideas:

1. **Maintain a Bedtime Pattern**
    - Going to bed and getting up at the same time each day can help the brain anticipate rest time.
    - This supports stable sleep cycles, which can improve memory and mood.
2. **Limit Evening Distractions**
    - Avoid watching intense or loud shows right before bed.
    - If worries keep you awake, write them down on a notepad next to your bed.
3. **Pre-Sleep Relaxation**
    - If you find yourself lying in bed awake, get up and do something calming, like reading or gentle stretching, until you feel sleepy again.
    - Going to bed only when you feel ready to rest can train the body to associate bed with sleep.
4. **Bedroom Comfort**
    - A comfortable mattress and pillows can improve sleep quality.
    - Keep the room cool and dimly lit for better rest.

Adequate sleep helps the brain recharge. Over time, good rest can make a real difference in how well you remember details and handle daily tasks.

Supporting Memory with Simple Techniques

Memory aids can make day-to-day life smoother. Some fresh suggestions include:

1. **Group Information**
   - When trying to remember several items, break them into groups. For example, if you have a shopping list, group fruits together, vegetables together, and so on.
2. **Link New Facts to Known Facts**
   - If you meet someone named "Rose," picture a rose flower next to her face in your mind.
   - Making a mental connection to something familiar can make details stick better.
3. **Use Rhymes or Silly Phrases**
   - For short bits of information, a quick rhyme might help.
   - It does not have to make sense to others, as long as it helps you recall something.
4. **Teach Others What You Know**
   - Explaining a recipe or an idea to a friend can reinforce it in your own mind.
   - The process of instructing someone else can make the information clearer in your head.
5. **Keep a Small Notebook**
   - Writing things down can help you remember, even if you never look at the note again.
   - The act of writing cements details in the mind.

Social Connections and Brain Function

Social interaction can boost mood, which helps the brain stay alert. Here are specific ways to mix social contact with mental stimulation:

1. **Group Discussions**
   - Meet with friends or neighbors to talk about a common interest, such as a movie you watched or a local issue.
   - Share ideas and ask questions to keep the conversation lively.
2. **Community Learning**

- Many places offer short, low-cost classes on arts, technology, or language.
    - Learning in a group can challenge the brain more than studying alone.
3. **Online Video Chats**
    - If you cannot meet in person, use simple video chat tools to connect with grandchildren or friends who live far away.
    - Share something small you learned that day and ask them about their day, too.
4. **Volunteer Work**
    - Volunteering can offer new experiences that keep the mind engaged.
    - Tasks like organizing items, greeting visitors, or helping with paperwork can all involve mental processes.

Being around people can sharpen thinking, as conversations often involve quick recall and adapting to new topics.

Foods That May Help the Brain

We have covered nutrition in earlier chapters, but here are some foods often linked to supporting the mind:

1. **Berries**
    - Blueberries, strawberries, and similar fruits have compounds that may help protect brain cells from stress.
    - Fresh, frozen, or dried berries can be part of meals or snacks.
2. **Leafy Greens**
    - Spinach, kale, and collard greens include vitamins and antioxidants.
    - They might help slow certain age-related mental changes.
3. **Nuts and Seeds**
    - Almonds, walnuts, flaxseeds, and chia seeds have healthy fats and nutrients that support overall brain function.
    - Try sprinkling seeds on oatmeal or salads for an easy boost.
4. **Whole Grains**
    - Oats, whole wheat, and brown rice provide a steady supply of energy for the brain.

- They also contain B vitamins, important for various body and brain processes.
5. **Fatty Fish**
    - Salmon, mackerel, and sardines supply omega-3 fatty acids, which may help keep brain cells healthy.
    - If you do not eat fish, talk to a medical professional about other sources or a supplement.

No single food can cure memory problems, but a balanced eating pattern with these choices can offer steady nourishment for the brain.

Avoiding Harmful Habits

Certain habits can harm the brain over time:

1. **Excessive Alcohol**
    - Drinking too much can affect memory and thinking.
    - If you choose to drink, do so in moderation according to your doctor's advice.
2. **Tobacco Use**
    - Smoking can harm blood flow, which is vital for brain health.
    - Quitting at any stage can help improve overall well-being.
3. **Chronic Sleep Loss**
    - Lack of consistent rest can lead to confusion and difficulty focusing.
    - Address sleep troubles as soon as they arise.
4. **Skipping Meals**
    - The brain needs steady fuel.
    - Extreme diets or missing meals might leave you feeling mentally fuzzy.
5. **Too Much Isolation**
    - Spending too much time alone can lead to mental dullness or sadness.
    - Connecting with others in small ways (phone calls, short visits) can brighten mood and thought processes.

Warning Signs of More Serious Brain Issues

It is normal to forget where you set your glasses. However, there can be signals that the problem is more than just age-related:

1. **Getting Lost in Familiar Places**
    - If you cannot find your way home on a route you know well, it could be a sign of bigger concerns.
2. **Forgetting Common Words Very Often**
    - Occasional slips happen, but frequent trouble with everyday words might need medical attention.
3. **Major Changes in Mood or Personality**
    - Sudden mood swings or behavior changes might indicate something more than normal aging.
4. **Trouble Following Steps**
    - For instance, if you can no longer follow a simple recipe or handle a task you used to do easily.
5. **Repeating Questions**
    - Asking the same question many times in a short period, not recalling you already asked, might be a sign of deeper memory problems.

If these appear, consider seeing a doctor. Sometimes, conditions like dementia or depression might affect how the brain functions. Early detection can lead to treatments or strategies that slow or manage symptoms.

Possible Medical and Professional Support

If you have ongoing concerns:

1. **Check-Ups**
    - Routine visits to a healthcare provider can catch any physical issues that might affect the brain, such as thyroid problems or vitamin deficiencies.
2. **Screenings**
    - Some clinics do simple tests to measure memory, language skills, or problem-solving.
    - These tests can spot areas that need attention.
3. **Counseling or Therapy**

- A counselor can help you handle fear or worry about memory loss.
- They can also teach strategies for coping with changes.
4. **Physical Therapy for Brain Health**
    - While it sounds odd, some physical therapists are trained in exercises that link body movements with mental tasks.
    - This can be especially helpful for older adults who want to stay sharp and steady on their feet.
5. **Community Resources**
    - Memory clinics or local support groups can offer insights for managing memory changes.
    - Sharing experiences with others in a similar situation can reduce feelings of being alone with the issue.

Brain-Friendly Daily Routines

1. **Structured Wake-Up and Wind-Down**
    - Start the day with a brief mental exercise, like recalling three positive things from the day before.
    - End the day by reviewing something you learned or a new thought you had.
2. **Midday Mental Boost**
    - After lunch, spend a few minutes challenging yourself mentally (like a word puzzle or a quick quiz).
    - This short burst can energize you during the afternoon slump.
3. **Rotate Hobbies**
    - If you like puzzles, do them for a while, then switch to listening to a short talk or engaging in a sketching exercise.
    - Changing tasks can spark different areas of the brain.
4. **Plan Simple Outings**
    - A short trip to a local museum or park can offer fresh sights and mental stimulation.
    - Just planning the outing (checking times, directions) is also a mental activity.
5. **Review the Day**
    - Before bed, think about what went well and one new thing you found interesting.
    - This reflection can help tie the day's memories together.

Digital Tools and the Brain

Smartphones, tablets, and computers can help or hinder brain health, depending on how they are used:

1. **Brain Training Apps**
    - Many apps offer short exercises that challenge memory, attention, or problem-solving.
    - Choose one that feels fun rather than frustrating.
2. **Online Classes**
    - You can find free classes on various subjects. Learning something new via short video lessons can keep your brain active.
    - Pick subjects you actually like to keep motivation high.
3. **Stay Balanced**
    - Too much screen time, especially on social media, can overwhelm the mind.
    - If you feel drained, step away from devices and do an offline activity.
4. **Use Reminders**
    - Set alarms or calendar alerts to help you remember important tasks (like medication times).
    - This frees mental space for other thoughts.

Encouraging a Positive Outlook

Worries about memory can create fear or sadness. Supporting a healthy mindset can help the brain function better:

1. **Note Progress**
    - If you learn a new trick—like how to use a new phone feature—acknowledge that you did it.
    - Giving yourself recognition can boost confidence in your abilities.
2. **Accept Imperfection**
    - Everyone forgets things sometimes. A small lapse does not mean you are failing.
    - Learning to laugh gently at a slip can reduce stress and help you move forward.
3. **Stay Open to Help**

- There is no shame in using lists, reminders, or asking people to repeat information.
- Let friends or relatives know you appreciate their patience.
4. **Keep Goals Realistic**
    - Setting huge mental challenges might be stressful. Choose modest goals that fit your comfort level.
    - Enjoy the feeling of mastering small tasks without pressuring yourself to be perfect.

Chapter Summary

- **Aging Brain Basics**: The brain can slow in certain areas, but it can still form new connections. Common memory concerns include losing items, forgetting names, and word-finding troubles.
- **Staying Mentally Engaged**: Mix up mental tasks, learn in small steps, and use recall exercises to boost memory. Everyday actions—like reading carefully or taking brief notes—can help strengthen the mind.
- **Healthy Routines**: Good sleep, balanced meals (with items like berries, leafy greens, nuts, seeds, whole grains, and fatty fish), and stress management support mental sharpness.
- **Warning Signs**: Major confusion or getting lost in familiar places may need medical attention. A doctor can run tests or suggest steps to manage more serious issues.
- **Practical Tools**: Use grouping techniques, mental links, short rhymes, or technology (like apps and reminders) to aid memory.
- **Positive Outlook**: Focus on small gains, accept slip-ups, and ask for help when needed. Socializing or volunteering can stimulate thinking and brighten mood.

By applying these fresh approaches, you can find it easier to handle normal memory lapses and keep your brain active. Even simple steps, like using new mental tasks or learning in small doses, can support a sharper mind. With a practical outlook and willingness to adapt, many older adults stay mentally agile and enjoy clear thinking in their everyday lives.

CHAPTER 8: EYE AND EAR CARE

Our eyes and ears let us see and hear the world around us. As people age, these senses can weaken, and that can change how we handle daily activities. Vision changes might involve difficulty reading small text or seeing well in dim light. Hearing loss can make it harder to follow conversations or enjoy music. In this chapter, we will explore how the eyes and ears can shift over time and offer practical tips to care for them. We will avoid repeating topics from earlier chapters, focusing instead on fresh guidance unique to these important senses.

Common Changes in Vision

1. **Presbyopia (Difficulty Focusing Up Close)**
   - Many people notice that small print or up-close tasks get harder, especially after age 40 or 50.
   - This happens because the eye's lens becomes less flexible, making it tougher to focus on nearby objects.
2. **Reduced Low-Light Vision**
   - Driving at dusk or seeing in a dimly lit room might become more challenging.
   - The pupils might not widen as much as before, limiting the light that enters the eye.
3. **Sensitivity to Glare**
   - Sunlight reflecting off water or shiny surfaces can be more intense.
   - This can cause discomfort or make it momentarily harder to see clearly.
4. **Cataracts**
   - The eye's lens can become cloudy over time, causing blurry or hazy vision.
   - Cataracts develop slowly, and many people do not notice them at first.
5. **Floaters**
   - Small specks or spots that drift across your field of view.
   - Often normal, but sudden increases might need a doctor's check.

Not every older adult will face all of these, but being aware can help you notice changes early and seek help if needed.

Tips for Protecting Vision

1. **Regular Eye Exams**
   - An eye doctor can spot issues like cataracts, glaucoma, or macular degeneration before they become severe.
   - They can also update your glasses or contact lens prescription to match changes in your eyesight.
2. **Use Proper Lighting**
   - When reading or doing detailed work, ensure there is enough light.
   - Position a lamp so it lights your task from behind or over your shoulder, preventing glare on the page.
3. **Wear Sunglasses**
   - Shades with 100% UV protection can reduce glare and shield the eyes from harmful rays.
   - A hat with a brim can also help protect eyes when outside.
4. **Take Breaks from Screens**
   - Staring at a phone, tablet, or computer for too long can lead to dry eyes and strain.
   - Follow the "20-20-20" rule: every 20 minutes, look at something about 20 feet away for 20 seconds.
5. **Be Mindful of Air Quality**
   - Dry air can irritate eyes. Use a humidifier if your home feels dry, especially in winter.
   - If you are in a dusty area, sunglasses or safety glasses might keep particles out.
6. **Choose Larger Text or Magnifiers**
   - If small print is a challenge, use large-print books or adjustable font sizes on devices.
   - Handheld magnifiers or reading glasses can reduce strain.
7. **Healthy Diet for Eyes**
   - Foods like carrots, sweet potatoes, spinach, and other colorful produce can supply vitamins A and C, along with other nutrients that support eye health.
   - Some research suggests fish rich in omega-3 fatty acids might also benefit vision.

Warning Signs for Vision Problems

Certain signs might point to something more serious:

1. **Sudden Blurriness or Blind Spots**
    - If vision changes happen quickly, see an eye doctor right away.
    - This might indicate a retinal problem or other serious issue.
2. **Intense Eye Pain or Redness**
    - Could be an infection or increased pressure inside the eye (glaucoma).
    - Seek urgent care if pain is severe or if you notice halos around lights.
3. **Double Vision**
    - Two images of a single object might suggest muscle or nerve concerns.
    - Even if it goes away, it is worth checking with a specialist.
4. **Loss of Peripheral Vision**
    - A gradual narrowing of your side vision can be linked to glaucoma.
    - It often appears so slowly that many people do not notice until it becomes advanced.

Early treatment can protect vision. Regular check-ups and quick attention to sudden changes can keep eyes healthier.

Low Vision Aids and Adjustments

For those with declining eyesight, certain tools or small changes can help:

1. **Magnifying Devices**
    - Besides reading glasses, handheld or stand magnifiers with built-in lights can enlarge text or details.
2. **Large-Print Materials**
    - Many libraries carry large-print versions of books and magazines.
    - Some digital devices let you increase font sizes for easier reading.
3. **Speech-to-Text Technology**
    - If reading text on a screen is tough, use apps that read out messages or online articles.
    - Many phones have built-in features to read text aloud.
4. **Enhanced Lighting**

- Nightlights in hallways or motion-sensor lights can help you move around safely.
- Under-cabinet lighting in the kitchen can make meal prep easier.

5. **High-Contrast Labels**
   - Using bright or bold labels on household items like spices or medication bottles can help you spot them quickly.
   - Keep backgrounds and text colors in high contrast (for instance, black text on a white label).
6. **Organized Living Spaces**
   - Keep walkways clear and furniture in consistent spots.
   - Use tactile markers (like raised dots or stickers) on important buttons (for example, stove knobs).

Low vision specialists can suggest more personalized aids and tips if your eyesight significantly decreases.

Common Hearing Changes with Age

1. **Presbycusis (Age-Related Hearing Loss)**
   - A slow loss of hearing, usually making higher-pitched sounds (like children's voices) harder to understand.
   - It can start gently and become more noticeable over time.
2. **Difficulty Following Conversations in Noisy Places**
   - Background noise (like in a restaurant) may make it tough to pick out words.
   - You might find yourself turning your ear toward a speaker or saying "What?" often.
3. **Tinnitus (Ringing in the Ears)**
   - A buzzing, ringing, or hissing sound in one or both ears.
   - Can be mild or sometimes bothersome enough to affect sleep or concentration.
4. **Reduced Sound Clarity**
   - Even if volume is loud enough, words may sound muffled.
   - Consonants like "s" or "t" might blend together.

Hearing loss is widespread among older adults, but many do not seek help, partly because changes happen slowly. Recognizing the signs can lead to better solutions.

Caring for Your Ears and Hearing

1. **Regular Hearing Checks**
   - If you notice signs of hearing loss or ringing in the ears, consider a hearing test.
   - An audiologist can measure hearing levels and suggest steps to manage or correct any loss.
2. **Limit Loud Noises**
   - Loud environments (like concerts or lawnmowing) can damage hearing further.
   - Use earplugs or noise-canceling headphones to protect your ears if you cannot avoid loud sounds.
3. **Turn Down the Volume**
   - When listening to music or TV, keep the volume at a safe level.
   - If someone next to you can clearly hear your headphones, it might be too loud.
4. **Avoid Sticking Objects in the Ear**
   - Cotton swabs or hairpins can injure the ear canal or eardrum.
   - If you have earwax problems, see a medical professional for safe removal.
5. **Watch for Ear Infections**
   - Signs might include pain, drainage, or sudden hearing changes.
   - Prompt care can prevent further damage.

Hearing Aids and Other Devices

If hearing loss affects daily life, hearing aids or assistive devices may help:

1. **Types of Hearing Aids**
   - Behind-the-ear (BTE): Sits behind the ear and connects to an earpiece.
   - In-the-ear (ITE): Fits in the outer ear area.
   - There are also smaller in-the-canal versions for mild to moderate loss.
2. **Choosing the Right Fit**
   - An audiologist will evaluate your type and degree of hearing loss, then recommend the style that suits you best.
   - Comfort is important, as you may wear it for many hours a day.

3. **Assistive Listening Devices**
    - TV amplifiers let you set a comfortable volume without turning the TV too loud for others.
    - Personal amplifiers use a small microphone and headphones, which can be handy in places with lots of background noise.
4. **Cochlear Implants**
    - For severe hearing loss, a cochlear implant bypasses damaged parts of the ear to deliver signals directly to the hearing nerve.
    - This is usually suggested when hearing aids are not enough, and it involves surgery plus follow-up therapy.

Hearing devices often require an adjustment period. Patience with new sounds and consistent use typically lead to better outcomes.

Communication Tips for Hearing Challenges

If you or someone near you has trouble hearing, these tips can make conversations clearer:

1. **Get Attention First**
    - Gently tap their shoulder or call their name before you start speaking.
    - Wait until they face you so they can read lips and expressions.
2. **Speak Clearly and Naturally**
    - Speak at a normal pace, but slightly louder if needed.
    - Avoid shouting or exaggerating mouth movements, as it can distort words.
3. **Eliminate Background Noise**
    - Turn off the TV or move away from noisy appliances before starting a conversation.
    - Sit closer to the person so your voice is easier to pick up.
4. **Rephrase Rather Than Repeat**
    - If they do not catch something, try saying it differently.
    - Sometimes certain words are harder to hear than others.
5. **Use Facial Expressions and Gestures**
    - Visual cues can help fill in gaps if words are missed.
    - Nodding, pointing, or showing an item can make the message clearer.

Preventing Further Hearing Damage

If you already have mild hearing loss:

1. **Mind Medication Side Effects**
    - Some drugs can worsen hearing problems. Ask your doctor if any of your prescriptions have this risk.
    - Never stop medication without talking to a professional, though—just be aware of possible effects.
2. **Stay Active**
    - Good circulation helps all parts of the body, including the ears.
    - Mild physical activity can support blood flow and overall health, though it is not a direct cure for hearing loss.
3. **Avoid Cigarette Smoke**
    - Being around tobacco smoke can harm hearing, as it affects blood vessels and nerves in the ear.
    - If you smoke, consider seeking help to stop.
4. **Manage Blood Pressure and Diabetes**
    - Conditions that affect blood flow can impact hearing.
    - Keep these under control with the help of your doctor to lower potential damage.

Balancing Eye and Ear Safety at Home

Small changes can make daily activities easier when vision or hearing is limited:

1. **Combine Visual and Audio Alerts**
    - Doorbells or alarms that flash lights as well as make noise can help if you have both hearing and sight changes.
    - Some telephones have bright visual ring signals.
2. **Label Important Sounds**
    - If certain beeps or alarms in your home are hard to hear, check if you can get devices that also vibrate or blink.
    - Smoke detectors and carbon monoxide alarms now come in versions for people with hearing loss.
3. **Clear Pathways**
    - If your vision is not as sharp, keep floors free of clutter to avoid trips.
    - Good lighting in key areas (like staircases) can reduce falls.

4. **Amplified Phones**
   - Some phones allow you to adjust volume or come with a built-in amplifier.
   - This makes phone calls easier if hearing is reduced.

Eye and Ear Friendly Hobbies

Hobbies can remain enjoyable with a few adaptations:

1. **Audiobooks or Podcasts**
   - If reading is getting tougher, consider listening to books.
   - Choose a volume and speed that are comfortable for you.
2. **Large-Scale Crafts**
   - If you enjoy crafting, use bigger needles or larger canvas patterns.
   - Good lighting and magnifying tools can help with fine details.
3. **Music with Visual Components**
   - If hearing is a challenge, choose videos where you can see the singer's face or read lyrics.
   - This allows you to follow along more easily.
4. **Social Games**
   - Card games with bigger fonts or board games with large pieces can be fun.
   - If hearing is an issue, consider quieter rooms or smaller groups.
5. **Nature Walks**
   - Walking outdoors can be relaxing.
   - If hearing is reduced, pay special attention to your surroundings for safety, or go with a companion who can help watch for hazards.

Seeing an Ear, Nose, and Throat Specialist (ENT)

If issues with your ears go beyond basic hearing loss, an ENT doctor might help:

1. **Ear Infections or Frequent Pain**
   - Chronic infections could damage the inner ear.
   - The ENT can diagnose and suggest treatments.
2. **Balance Problems**

- The inner ear helps with balance. If you often feel dizzy or unsteady, there might be an inner ear cause.
- Tests can pinpoint whether it is an ear-related balance issue.
3. **Unusual Discharge**
    - Fluids coming from the ear might signal infection or injury.
    - An ENT can find the reason and give proper care.
4. **Tinnitus Management**
    - If ringing in the ears is severe, the ENT may suggest therapies or sound-masking devices to ease the discomfort.

Eye and Ear Checklists

Here are brief checklists to keep track of eye and ear care:

- **Eye Care**
    - Yearly or bi-yearly eye exams
    - Proper lighting in rooms
    - Sunglasses with UV protection
    - Follow the "20-20-20" rule for screens
    - Watch for sudden vision changes
    - Use magnifiers or large print if needed
- **Ear Care**
    - Hearing checks if you notice changes
    - Avoid loud noises or use earplugs
    - Keep volumes moderate
    - Watch for signs of infection or pain
    - Consider hearing aids or devices if recommended
    - Maintain healthy blood pressure and limit smoking exposure

Keeping these items in mind can guide you toward better sensory health.

Emotional Side of Vision and Hearing Changes

Losing some vision or hearing can affect how we feel. You might worry about safety or feel left out in group conversations. Here are ways to handle the emotional impact:

1. **Communicate Feelings**
    - Talk with friends or family about frustrations.
    - Sometimes they can adjust how they interact to help you feel included.
2. **Find Support Groups**
    - Local or online communities can share tips for living with hearing or vision loss.
    - Learning from people who understand your situation can be encouraging.
3. **Boost Independence**
    - Practice using new tools (like magnifiers or hearing aids) until you feel more confident.
    - Overcoming small obstacles can lift your mood.
4. **Seek Professional Guidance**
    - Counselors or therapists can help if sadness or anxiety become overwhelming.
    - They can teach coping techniques or connect you with resources.

Remember, many older adults face similar difficulties, so you are not alone. Reaching out can bring fresh ideas and a sense of comfort.

CHAPTER 9: PROTECTING SKIN AND HAIR

Our skin is our body's outer layer. It shields us from germs, helps regulate body temperature, and gives us our sense of touch. Hair, on the other hand, can protect the scalp from sunlight and offer warmth for the head. As people get older, both skin and hair often change. Skin might become thinner or drier, and hair can turn gray and become more fragile. In this chapter, we will look at why these changes happen and how to care for skin and hair in ways that fit older age. We will share new ideas specific to skin and hair, without repeating tips we have covered before.

Why Skin and Hair Change Over Time

1. **Less Collagen and Elasticity**
    - Collagen is a protein that supports the skin's structure. It can start to break down with age, making the skin thinner and less firm.
    - Elastic fibers in the skin become weaker, leading to more wrinkles.
2. **Lower Oil Production**
    - Oil glands in the skin can slow down, causing dryness.
    - Dry skin may peel, crack, or become itchy if not cared for properly.
3. **Sun Damage Build-Up**
    - Over the years, sunlight can cause changes like age spots (flat, brown patches) and wrinkles.
    - The sun's rays can also affect hair, making it more brittle or changing its texture.
4. **Hair Pigment Changes**
    - Gray or white hairs appear as pigment cells in the hair reduce.
    - Some people notice thinning hair or a change in hair's thickness or texture.
5. **Hormonal Shifts**
    - After certain life phases, like menopause in women, hormones that once supported hair growth and skin oils adjust.
    - This can lead to hair thinning and a drier skin surface.

Everyone's skin and hair will age in unique ways, partly due to genetics and partly from habits like sun exposure and nutrition. Even though we cannot stop time, we can help skin and hair stay healthier longer with consistent care.

Simple Ways to Protect and Nourish Skin

1. **Gentle Cleansing**
   - Use mild soaps or cleansers that do not strip the skin of its natural oils.
   - Avoid very hot water; lukewarm water is kinder to aging skin.
2. **Moisturizing**
   - Apply a fragrance-free moisturizer on damp skin right after bathing.
   - Look for products that contain ingredients like glycerin, ceramides, or hyaluronic acid to help lock in moisture.
3. **Avoid Harsh Scrubbing**
   - Exfoliating can remove dead skin cells, but do so gently.
   - Rough scrubs or strong brushes may irritate thin, sensitive skin.
4. **Protect Against Irritants**
   - Wear gloves when doing chores that involve chemicals (like cleaning products) to prevent dryness or rashes.
   - If you notice new redness or itching after using a product, discontinue it and see if symptoms improve.
5. **Sun Protection**
   - Applying sunscreen (SPF 30 or higher) can help reduce future wrinkles and age spots.
   - If you spend time outdoors, consider wearing a broad-brimmed hat and lightweight, long-sleeved clothing.
6. **Stay Hydrated**
   - Drinking enough water supports overall skin health.
   - While water alone will not completely prevent dryness, it helps maintain normal skin function alongside other protective steps.
7. **Use a Humidifier**
   - If indoor air is dry (often during winter), a humidifier can add moisture to the environment.
   - This can help lessen skin dryness and irritation.

Addressing Common Skin Concerns

1. **Itching and Dry Spots**
   - Older skin can become itchy. Moisturizing often and using gentle soaps can help soothe dryness.

- Wearing soft, breathable fabrics (like cotton) can minimize friction on itchy areas.
2. **Age Spots and Uneven Tone**
    - These are often linked to sun exposure over many years.
    - While they are not usually harmful, you can check with a dermatologist if you see any changing spots.
    - Some over-the-counter creams aim to lighten dark patches, but results vary.
3. **Bruising and Thin Skin**
    - With thinning skin, bumps can lead to bruises that appear larger or more colorful than before.
    - Protective clothing (like long sleeves) and being gentle when handling the skin can help lower bruising.
4. **Pressure Sores**
    - People who spend a lot of time in bed or sitting in one spot can develop sores on bony areas.
    - Regularly changing position and using cushions can reduce this risk.
5. **Skin Tags or Growths**
    - Small, harmless growths can appear with age. If they bother you or change shape, a doctor can remove them.
    - Keep an eye on any spot that changes color, size, or shape quickly, as it could signal a more serious issue.

If you notice any new or unusual changes in moles or spots, it is always best to consult a healthcare professional for an exam. Early detection is key for skin health.

Hair Care for Older Adults

1. **Use Mild Shampoos**
    - Pick shampoos labeled "gentle" or "for dry hair." Avoid harsh formulas that can remove oils from the scalp.
    - Too much shampooing can dry out hair, so aim for a routine that keeps hair clean yet not stripped of moisture (this varies by person).
2. **Condition Regularly**

- A creamy conditioner can replenish moisture and help detangle hair.
- If hair is very dry, leave-in conditioners or hair oils (like argan oil) can add softness.

3. **Avoid Tight Hairstyles**
   - Pulling hair back strongly (like in tight ponytails or braids) may lead to tension on the scalp and further thinning.
   - Opt for looser styles or gentle clips that do not tug at the hair roots.
4. **Gentle Combing**
   - Use a wide-tooth comb or a soft brush. Start from the ends to ease out tangles, then move up.
   - Being too rough can break fragile hair.
5. **Manage Heat Styling**
   - Curling irons, straighteners, and blow dryers may weaken hair, especially if used often or at high heat.
   - Consider air-drying or using low-heat settings if possible. A heat-protective spray can also reduce damage.
6. **Cut and Style for Comfort**
   - A shorter haircut can make thin hair look fuller, and it is often simpler to care for.
   - Ask a hairstylist for tips on flattering cuts that work well with changing hair textures.
7. **Handling Gray or White Hair**
   - Gray hair can be more coarse or dry, so extra conditioning might be helpful.
   - If you choose to color your hair, pick gentle dyes or consider professional help to minimize hair shaft damage.

Scalp Health and Hair Loss

Hair thinning can come from several causes, including genetics, hormonal changes, or certain medications. Here are steps to support scalp health:

1. **Scalp Checks**
   - Gently feel your scalp for any bumps, dryness, or irritation.
   - Let a doctor know if you notice red patches or sores that do not heal.

2. **Dandruff Control**
    - Dandruff (white flakes) can be managed with shampoos that contain zinc pyrithione or other anti-dandruff agents.
    - If it does not improve, a dermatologist can suggest stronger treatments.
3. **Avoid Over-Brushing**
    - Some people believe brushing hair 100 times daily is helpful, but too much friction can break fragile strands.
    - A light daily brushing is enough to distribute natural oils without overdoing it.
4. **Medicated Products**
    - If hair loss is significant, certain over-the-counter topical treatments (like minoxidil) might slow it.
    - Your doctor can guide you on whether these are safe and which product is best.
5. **Balanced Nutrition**
    - Nutrients like protein, iron, and certain vitamins support hair growth.
    - If you have diet restrictions, ask a healthcare professional about supplements that may help.

Hair loss can be emotional, but there are options like different haircuts, gentle coloring, or even wigs that some individuals find to be good solutions. The most important thing is to keep the scalp comfortable and the hair that remains as healthy as possible.

Tips for Sun Protection (Skin and Hair)

While we touched on basic sun protection before, let's add more detail:

1. **Broad-Spectrum Sunscreen**
    - Look for "broad-spectrum" on the label. This means it protects from both UVA (aging rays) and UVB (burning rays).
    - Apply sunscreen at least 15 minutes before going outside and reapply every two hours or after sweating or swimming.
2. **Sun-Protective Clothing**
    - Some clothing lines offer fabrics with built-in UV protection.
    - Wide hats can shade the face, neck, and scalp. This is especially helpful if hair is thin or parted.

3. **Lip Balm with SPF**
   - Lips can also be harmed by the sun. Use a lip balm that has SPF to prevent dryness and cracking.
   - Reapply when you feel it is wearing off.
4. **Protecting the Scalp**
   - If you have thinning hair, your scalp might get sunburned easily.
   - Apply sunscreen on exposed scalp areas or wear a head covering.
5. **Timing**
   - The sun's rays are strongest midday (usually between 10 a.m. and 4 p.m.).
   - If possible, plan outdoor tasks for earlier or later in the day to avoid the highest UV exposure.

By combining these steps, you not only lower the risk of sunburn and further skin aging, but you also help keep hair from drying out in intense sunlight.

Watching for Skin Changes Linked to Health

Skin can show signs of underlying conditions:

1. **Dry, Flaky Patches**
   - Sometimes, very dry patches can point to thyroid issues or other imbalances.
   - If dryness is severe and not improving with moisturizers, it might be worth checking with a doctor.
2. **Yellowish Skin or Eyes**
   - This can suggest problems with the liver, such as jaundice.
   - Seek medical guidance if you notice a sudden change in skin tone.
3. **Nails**
   - While nails are not exactly skin, they are related. Brittle or ridged nails could indicate nutrition concerns.
   - If nails become thick, discolored, or painful, you might have a fungal infection or other issue.
4. **Slow Wound Healing**
   - If small cuts or scrapes take a very long time to heal, it might point to issues like diabetes or poor circulation.
   - Keep any wound clean, watch for signs of infection, and check with a healthcare professional if it does not improve.
5. **Swelling or Fluid Retention**

- Changes in the skin around the ankles or feet, like swelling, could indicate circulation or kidney problems.

Being aware of these signs can help you catch and treat health concerns early. Of course, only a medical professional can diagnose the cause, but observing skin changes is a good starting point.

Pampering Skin Safely

A little pampering can boost comfort and help older skin look and feel better:

1. **Mild Baths or Soaks**
   - Adding oatmeal or special bath oils can soothe itchy, dry skin.
   - Keep the water temperature warm, not hot, to avoid stripping oils.
2. **Face Masks**
   - Look for calming masks with gentle ingredients like aloe vera or cucumber extract if you enjoy that spa feel.
   - Avoid harsh peeling masks that might irritate sensitive skin.
3. **Hand and Foot Care**
   - Soaking feet in warm water softens calluses. Follow with a foot cream.
   - Hands might need extra moisturizer, especially after washing dishes or gardening.
4. **Professional Treatments**
   - A licensed esthetician with experience caring for older skin can offer gentle facials or other treatments.
   - Always mention any medical conditions or sensitivities before a spa visit.

Pampering is not just about appearance. Caring for the skin can help prevent dryness, cracks, or minor infections that arise from neglected skin.

Possible Skin Therapies and Medications

If dryness, rashes, or other concerns do not improve with basic care, a doctor might suggest:

1. **Prescription Creams**
   - Some contain steroids for redness or itching, while others may have stronger moisturizers for chronic dryness.
   - Use them exactly as instructed, as overuse can thin the skin further or cause other side effects.
2. **Medicated Shampoos**
   - These can control scalp conditions like psoriasis or severe dandruff.
   - Follow directions carefully, since some products must stay on the scalp for a set time before rinsing.
3. **Light Therapy**
   - Under medical supervision, certain skin problems may improve with controlled light (like UVB for psoriasis).
   - This is usually done in a clinic to ensure safe exposure.
4. **Laser Treatments**
   - In some cases, doctors use lasers to treat age spots or certain growths.
   - This is often for cosmetic reasons but can also help remove early-stage skin problems.
5. **Oral Medications**
   - If a skin issue is linked to infection or inflammation inside the body, oral drugs might help.
   - Always review possible side effects and interactions with your doctor.

Remember that every treatment comes with considerations. Balancing the benefits with any risks is important, and a qualified healthcare professional can guide you in making informed choices.

Dealing with Minor Skin Infections

Older skin can be more prone to small infections. Here are steps to avoid or handle them:

1. **Keep Cuts Clean**
   - Even minor nicks can let germs in. Rinse with mild soap and water, then pat dry.
   - Cover with a clean bandage if the area is in contact with clothing or dirt.

2. **Watch for Redness or Swelling**
   - If the skin around a cut becomes red, hot, or starts oozing fluid, it might be infected.
   - Seek medical help if symptoms get worse or do not improve with basic care.
3. **Foot Care**
   - Moisture between toes can lead to fungal problems like athlete's foot.
   - Dry feet thoroughly after bathing and wear breathable socks.
4. **Fungal Nail Infections**
   - Nails might look thicker, yellowish, or crumble at the edges.
   - Over-the-counter antifungal treatments exist, but severe cases may need prescription medication.
5. **Check Shoes for Fit**
   - Ill-fitting shoes can cause blisters that might become infected, especially if you have circulation problems.
   - Ensure your toes are not cramped and that there is some wiggle room.

Minor infections can often be treated at home if caught early. For deeper or persistent infections, professional care is essential.

Healthy Habits for Skin and Hair from Within

We have covered external steps, but internal factors also matter:

1. **Stay Hydrated**
   - We mentioned water intake earlier, but it bears repeating: consistent fluid intake supports normal skin function.
   - If you have kidney or heart conditions, follow a doctor's advice on fluid limits.
2. **Eat Balanced Meals**
   - Vitamin C (in citrus fruits, bell peppers) can support collagen production.
   - Lean proteins (like chicken, beans, or fish) help build the building blocks for hair and skin cells.
3. **Watch Sugar and Highly Processed Foods**
   - Some studies suggest high sugar intake can speed up skin aging by affecting collagen.

     - Whole, minimally processed foods may help keep blood sugar steady and skin healthier.
 4. **Get Enough Rest**
     - Sleep is when the body repairs and renews cells, including those in the skin.
     - Aim for a regular sleep schedule if possible, as restless nights can lead to dull skin and dryness.
 5. **Manage Stress**
     - High stress can sometimes trigger skin issues like flare-ups of eczema or hair thinning.
     - We will cover stress in more detail in the next chapter, but it is helpful to know that calm routines can benefit your skin and hair, too.

Hair Styling Alternatives

If thinning hair is a concern, here are some style ideas:

 1. **Layered Cuts**
     - Layers add volume, making hair look fuller.
     - Shorter layers around the face can also draw attention away from thin spots.
 2. **Wigs or Hairpieces**
     - Modern options can look natural and can be worn occasionally or daily.
     - Proper fitting is key to comfort.
 3. **Scarves or Hats**
     - Colorful scarves, headbands, or hats can be both stylish and protective against sun.
     - Lightweight materials help avoid overheating the scalp.
 4. **Hair Fibers**
     - Some products, like keratin hair fibers, can cling to existing strands, giving the look of thicker hair.
     - They wash out easily with shampoo.

Choosing a method depends on personal comfort. Some prefer to embrace gray or thinning hair, while others enjoy exploring style changes. The goal is to feel comfortable and confident.

Checking In with a Dermatologist

A dermatologist specializes in skin, hair, and nails. Reasons to see one include:

- **Persistent Rashes or Itching**
  If dryness or itchiness will not go away, a dermatologist can find the cause.
- **Suspicious Moles or Growths**
  Early checks can catch serious conditions like skin cancer.
- **Severe Hair Loss**
  They might spot an underlying cause and guide possible treatments.
- **Specific Cosmetic Concerns**
  For instance, professional treatments for deep wrinkles or age spots.

Dermatologists can offer tailored advice and treatments that fit an older adult's health needs.

CHAPTER 10: HANDLING STRESS IN OLDER AGE

Many people feel stressed at times, no matter their stage in life. However, older adults can face unique stressors like health concerns, changes in independence, or shifts in living arrangements. While a bit of stress can push us to solve problems, too much over a long period can lead to fatigue, worry, or even health issues. In this chapter, we will look at fresh ways to manage stress that do not repeat our earlier guidance on general well-being. We will focus on practical ideas suited to older adults seeking steady calmness.

Why Stress Can Feel Different in Older Age

1. **Life Transitions**
    - Retirement can shift daily routines, leaving some individuals feeling uncertain about how to fill their time.
    - Downsizing or moving to a different home might create emotional strain.
2. **Health Concerns**
    - Chronic pain, new medical diagnoses, or caring for a spouse with health problems can add worry.
    - The body may not handle stress hormones as easily as it once did, leading to a heightened sense of tension.
3. **Social Changes**
    - Friends or family may move away, and social circles can become smaller. Loneliness itself can trigger stress or sadness.
    - Feeling isolated can make everyday challenges more overwhelming.
4. **Financial Worries**
    - Living on a fixed income can create concern about bills or unexpected costs.
    - Changes in healthcare needs may also raise money-related stress.

Understanding these differences can help older adults seek methods that bring relief and fit their current life stage.

Physical Effects of Long-Term Stress

Chronic stress does not just affect emotions; it can affect the body:

1. **Higher Blood Pressure**
    - Stress hormones might cause spikes in blood pressure, which could strain the heart over time.
    - While brief changes are normal, ongoing high blood pressure poses a health risk.
2. **Tense Muscles**
    - Shoulders, neck, and back may feel tight or painful if stress becomes a habit.
    - Headaches can also appear due to muscle tension in the scalp or neck.
3. **Sleep Troubles**
    - Stress can make it harder to fall asleep or stay asleep, leading to tiredness the next day.
    - Ongoing lack of rest can impact concentration, mood, and overall health.
4. **Weakened Immune Response**
    - Some studies suggest that too much stress for too long may reduce the body's ability to fight off infections.
    - Older adults might feel the impact more if they already have other health conditions.
5. **Digestive Upset**
    - Stress can lead to an upset stomach, reduced appetite, or changes in bowel habits.
    - Focusing on mild meals and stress-lowering tips may help balance digestion.

Recognizing these signs as stress-related can help you realize when you need to ease tension and seek healthier coping methods.

Quick Tension Breakers

Sometimes stress builds up during the day. Here are short actions to interrupt stress before it grows:

1. **Focused Sigh**

- Take a deep breath, then let it out slowly with a long sighing sound.
    - A few mindful sighs can reset the pace of breathing and reduce tension in the shoulders.
2. **Shoulder Rolls**
    - Roll shoulders forward five times, then backward five times.
    - This loosens tight muscles and refreshes circulation in the upper back.
3. **Spot Relaxation**
    - Pick one area, like your forehead or hands, and consciously relax the muscles there for 10 seconds.
    - Move to a different area, like your jaw or feet, and do the same. Gradually, the body feels calmer.
4. **Soft Music Break**
    - Listen to a calming tune for one minute, focusing on the melody rather than your worries.
    - If music is not your preference, try nature sounds like gentle rain or birdsong.
5. **Phone a Positive Contact**
    - If you can call someone who offers support or good humor, a brief chat can pull your mind away from stress.
    - Even a couple of minutes can improve mood.

These mini-breaks are easy to slip into a routine. They can also serve as reminders that you have some control over moments of tension.

Building a Regular Calm Routine

Some stress management works best when practiced consistently. Consider adding these habits to daily life:

1. **Light Stretching Upon Waking**
    - Before getting out of bed, gently stretch arms and legs. Roll ankles and wrists in circles.
    - This signals the body to move gently into the day rather than rushing.
2. **Mid-Day Pause**
    - Schedule a short period (maybe after lunch) to sit quietly or do a calm activity, like simple knitting or easy puzzles.

- Think of it as a reset button during your day.
3. **Pre-Bed Wind-Down**
   - Avoid intense news or social media right before bedtime.
   - Instead, read a calming book, listen to soothing music, or write in a small notebook about the day's positives.
4. **Mental Organization**
   - At a set time each day, note important tasks or concerns on paper.
   - Putting them on a list may free your mind from holding everything in, reducing mental clutter.
5. **Gentle Hobbies**
   - Activities like painting with watercolors, tending to potted plants, or working on a small model can be relaxing.
   - Pick something that absorbs your attention without feeling like a chore.

Having a predictable routine helps the body and mind anticipate calm moments, reducing overall stress levels.

Handling Stress from Health Changes

1. **Clear Communication with Doctors**
   - If your medical condition causes worry, ask questions during appointments until you understand the situation.
   - Being informed can relieve fear of the unknown.
2. **Break Down Care Plans**
   - If you have multiple care steps (like taking meds, doing physical therapy), list them in an order that feels manageable.
   - Celebrate (or rather, acknowledge) each small success instead of focusing on the entire plan at once.
3. **Seek Support**
   - If you need rides to the doctor or help with errands, let family or friends know.
   - Feeling alone in handling health can heighten stress, so leaning on a support system can lessen the load.
4. **Gentle Movement Options**
   - If your mobility is limited, seated exercises or simple arm lifts can still help relieve tension.

- Consult a physical therapist for custom routines that fit your condition.
5. **Focus on What You Can Do**
    - Sometimes, stress arises from dwelling on what used to be easy.
    - Adjust tasks if needed. For instance, if standing too long is painful, sit on a stool to cook or fold laundry.

Emotional Resilience Tips

Emotional resilience is the ability to adapt when facing difficulties. It does not mean ignoring problems, but rather finding balanced ways to handle them:

1. **Give Yourself Credit**
    - Acknowledge the challenges you have already overcome. This self-awareness can inspire confidence for future hurdles.
    - Remind yourself: "I managed tough times before; I can handle new ones, too."
2. **Look for Humor**
    - While life is serious at times, seeking small moments of humor can lighten stress.
    - Whether it is a funny TV show, a silly memory, or a chat with a witty friend, laughter can ease tension.
3. **Adjust Expectations**
    - If you find certain tasks (like heavy housework) too demanding, consider scaling back or requesting help.
    - Setting realistic goals can prevent frustration.
4. **Practice Self-Compassion**
    - Speak to yourself the way you would speak to a friend in need: with kindness and understanding.
    - Accept that everyone has limits and that slowing down is part of normal aging.
5. **Limit Negative News**
    - Constant exposure to troubling news can worsen stress.
    - Stay informed, but choose how much time you spend on difficult topics.

Mindful Approaches Without Complexity

Some mindful practices can be simple, requiring no special training:

1. **Five Senses Check-In**
   - Pause and notice at least one thing you can see, hear, feel, smell, and (if appropriate) taste around you.
   - This brings your mind to the present moment, easing worries about past or future.
2. **Gentle Counting**
   - Close your eyes (if it is safe) and count your breaths up to 10, then start again.
   - If thoughts wander, gently bring attention back to the count without judgment.
3. **Visual Comfort**
   - Look at something pleasant for a short while: a flower, a favorite photo, or a calming view.
   - Simply observe details, like colors or shapes, without trying to analyze them.
4. **Hand-On-Heart Pause**
   - Place a hand on your heart or chest area and notice the warmth, your heartbeat, or rising and falling of the breath.
   - This small touch can feel comforting and remind you to slow down for a moment.
5. **Listening to Calm Beats**
   - If music resonates with you, find a slow rhythm or instrumental piece.
   - Focus on each note or instrument as it unfolds, preventing your mind from racing to worries.

None of these techniques need specialized equipment or extensive knowledge. They serve as mental anchors in your day, grounding you when tension arises.

Social Stress and Ways to Cope

Sometimes stress comes from interactions with others:

1. **Set Boundaries**

- If phone calls with certain people leave you frazzled, consider limiting the length of these calls or scheduling them when you feel calmest.
- Communicate kindly about your need for shorter or less frequent chats if they become too draining.

2. **Plan Small Gatherings**
    - Large group events might be noisy or overwhelming. Instead, invite one or two friends for tea or a simple meal.
    - This allows for relaxed conversation without much stress.
3. **Use Written Communication**
    - If misunderstandings happen often in spoken conversations, writing letters or emails can give you time to choose words carefully.
    - It also gives the other person space to process before responding.
4. **Seek Mediation if Needed**
    - If family conflicts arise, a neutral counselor or trusted friend might help bridge misunderstandings.
    - A calm environment can encourage everyone to listen rather than argue.
5. **Stay Connected with Positive People**
    - A sense of community lowers stress. Focus on those who offer kind support.
    - Even quick chats with neighbors or seeing familiar faces at a local store can boost spirits.

Fun Activities for Stress Relief

Finding joy in small ways can counter stress:

1. **Low-Key Arts**
    - Painting, drawing, or coloring books can be soothing. They do not require you to be an expert—just enjoy the process.
    - Finger paints (designed for adults) are another playful option if you want to free your creative side without worry.
2. **Gentle Drumming**
    - Tapping a simple beat on a table or drum might release tension.
    - Even small percussive movements can be calming if done at a slow tempo.

3. **Story Sharing**
   - Record personal memories or stories in a journal or on an audio device.
   - This can bring back pleasant times and a sense of legacy, easing stress by focusing on meaningful experiences.
4. **Puzzles and Board Games**
   - Solo puzzles like crosswords or jigsaws are engaging but not stressful if you take your time.
   - Playing a simple board game with a friend or family member can shift attention away from worries.
5. **Nature Connection**
   - If possible, sit by a window to watch birds or plant a small flower in a pot.
   - Observing living things can induce calm and ground you in the present.

The key is to pick hobbies or pastimes you genuinely enjoy, rather than forcing yourself into something that feels like a chore.

When to Seek Professional Help

While personal coping strategies can handle mild stress, consider professional support if:

1. **Stress Interferes with Daily Life**
   - If you cannot complete normal tasks due to worry or tension, it might be time to talk with a counselor.
   - Not being able to sleep or eat properly can be a sign stress is too high.
2. **Feelings of Hopelessness or Sadness**
   - If you have ongoing low mood or a sense that nothing will improve, a mental health professional can help.
   - Older adults can experience depression that looks like constant fatigue or lack of interest in usual activities.
3. **Panic Attacks**
   - Sudden periods of intense fear, racing heart, or feeling unable to breathe are serious.
   - A therapist can teach specific skills to handle and lessen these attacks.

4. **Chronic Pain or Physical Symptoms Linked to Stress**
   - Sometimes body aches or stomach troubles persist if the root cause is anxiety.
   - Doctors and therapists can work together to find solutions.
5. **Need for Medication**
   - In some cases, short-term medication can help manage intense anxiety or depression while you learn coping tools.
   - Always discuss pros and cons with a doctor to ensure it fits your health profile.

Seeking help is a sign of strength. Support from a professional can bring fresh strategies or uncover underlying issues that you might not spot alone.

Additional Resources

- **Support Groups**: Local community centers or senior organizations may host groups where peers share tips and offer emotional support.
- **Online Platforms**: Some websites or apps provide guided relaxation or calming exercises at no or low cost.
- **Local Help Lines**: Many places have hotlines for older adults who need someone to talk to about stress or loneliness.

Asking about these options at a clinic or library might reveal services you did not know were available.

CHAPTER 11: SLEEP TIPS FOR BETTER REST

Sleep is a basic need that helps our minds and bodies work at their best. It can affect how much energy we have, how we feel, and even how strong our immune system is. Many older adults find it harder to sleep well through the night. They might wake up often or feel groggy in the morning. Getting enough rest is important, even if our sleep patterns shift over time. In this chapter, we will look at factors that affect sleep in older age, share ideas for improving bedtime routines and the bedroom environment, and offer suggestions to help you fall asleep and stay asleep without repeating advice from earlier chapters.

Why Sleep Might Change in Later Years

1. **Shift in Internal Clock**
    - Each person has a "body clock," also known as the circadian rhythm. As people age, this rhythm can move earlier, causing them to feel tired sooner in the evening and wake up before sunrise.
    - This might not match the sleep schedule a person had when they were younger, leading to confusion about why they cannot stay asleep until morning.
2. **Lighter Sleep Stages**
    - During sleep, the body cycles through stages: light sleep, deeper sleep, and periods of dreaming (REM sleep). Older adults might spend less time in the deeper stages of sleep, meaning they can wake up more easily from small noises or discomfort.
    - This can lead to feeling less rested, even if the total number of hours in bed seems the same as before.
3. **Medical Concerns**
    - Health conditions such as arthritis or heartburn can cause nighttime discomfort. People might also need to use the bathroom more often, interrupting sleep.
    - Some medications can disrupt rest, either by causing drowsiness during the day or making it hard to relax at night.
4. **Reduced Daytime Activity**
    - If a person is less active during the day, the body might not feel the need for as much nighttime recovery.
    - Spending a lot of time seated can also lead to daytime dozing, which can spoil nighttime rest if naps run too long.

5. **Stress or Worry**
    - Older adults might face anxieties about health, finances, or family. These concerns can fill the mind and make it difficult to relax at bedtime.
    - When thoughts race, the body might stay in a more alert state, delaying sleep.

Recognizing these potential reasons for changing sleep helps us find better methods to rest. Not everyone will face the same issues, but many older adults notice at least some shifts in their sleep patterns.

Setting Up the Bedroom for Better Sleep

1. **Keep It Cool and Comfortable**
    - A cool room, around 65 to 70 degrees Fahrenheit, often helps with deeper sleep.
    - Bedding that is too warm can lead to sweating and discomfort, so layering blankets can be handy. That way, you can remove layers if you get too hot.
2. **Limit Light**
    - Darkness tells the body it is time to rest. Use heavy curtains or blinds to block outside lights, such as street lamps or passing car headlights.
    - A small nightlight in the hallway or bathroom can help you move around safely if you need to get up without filling the bedroom with bright light.
3. **Reduce Noise**
    - A quiet room reduces the chance of being awakened by random sounds. If you cannot control outside noise, consider earplugs or a simple sound machine that plays gentle background noise.
    - Some people use a small fan that produces a steady, soft hum, which can mask sudden sounds like distant traffic.
4. **Comfortable Mattress and Pillows**
    - A supportive mattress helps older joints feel better during the night. If a mattress is too firm or too soft, it can lead to back or hip discomfort.
    - Pillows come in various shapes and materials, so finding one that supports your neck can make a big difference in waking up with fewer aches.

5. **Avoid Screen Glare**
    - Televisions, tablets, or phones emit a type of light that can trick the brain into thinking it is daytime.
    - If you like reading before bed, consider using a small bedside lamp rather than a bright overhead light. If you use a reading device, lower the brightness or shift it to a warmer, dimmer setting.
6. **Safe Pathways**
    - If you need to use the bathroom during the night, ensure the path is clear of clutter or loose rugs. A small motion-sensor light can guide the way without blasting the room with brightness.
    - This helps prevent falls and the stress of stumbling in the dark.

Bedtime Routines for Deeper Rest

1. **Wind Down Early**
    - Give yourself 30 to 60 minutes before bedtime to slow down. Avoid high-energy activities like sorting out finances or watching loud action shows.
    - Soft music, gentle stretches, or warm (not hot) showers can calm the body.
2. **Set a Regular Schedule**
    - Going to bed and getting up at the same time each day can help the body's internal clock.
    - Even on weekends, try to stay close to your usual routine so you do not confuse your sleep-wake cycle.
3. **Limit Late-Day Caffeine**
    - Caffeine can stay in the system for hours, so having coffee or strong tea in the late afternoon might keep you awake at night.
    - Try switching to herbal teas or water by mid-afternoon, especially if you are sensitive to caffeine's effects.
4. **Keep Evening Meals Light**
    - Heavy or spicy dinners can lead to indigestion or heartburn when lying down.
    - If you get hungry at night, have a small snack such as a piece of toast or some fruit. Avoid big servings of sugary or fatty foods that might unsettle the stomach.
5. **Check Medications**
    - Some pills, like certain decongestants or steroids, can make it hard to relax. Others might cause nighttime bathroom trips if they act as diuretics.

- If your bedtime routine is constantly disrupted, ask your doctor if an adjustment in dosage timing is possible.
6. **Keep the Bed for Sleep**
    - If you spend a lot of time in bed browsing on a laptop or phone, your body might associate the bed with staying awake.
    - Use the bed mostly for sleep. That way, when you lie down, the mind connects that action with rest.

Exercises and Stretches That May Help Sleep

Though we spoke about physical activity in earlier chapters, here are some fresh, simple moves specifically aimed at relaxing the body before bed:

1. **Seated Forward Bend (in a Chair)**
    - Sit on a chair with feet flat on the floor. Slowly fold your upper body forward, letting arms dangle. Breathe quietly for a few slow counts, then lift your body upright again. This can stretch the lower back and loosen the shoulders.
2. **Slow Neck Rolls**
    - Gently tilt your head toward one shoulder, circle forward, then toward the other shoulder, and finally back to the starting spot. Move very slowly and stop if you feel pain. Neck rolls can release tension from the day.
3. **Leg Extensions**
    - Sit or lie down on your back and extend one leg gently, pointing your toes. Then relax and switch legs. This helps the legs and feet calm down, especially if they are restless.
4. **Deep Belly Breathing**
    - Place a hand on your abdomen. Inhale slowly through your nose, feeling your abdomen rise. Exhale gently through your mouth and feel your abdomen fall.
    - Repeat for a few minutes, aiming to keep each breath smooth and steady.
5. **Progressive Muscle Tensing and Releasing**
    - Starting from your toes, tense the muscles in your feet, hold for a moment, then release. Move upwards to your calves, thighs, and so on up to your face.
    - This step-by-step method can help you notice and release areas that might still be tight from the day.

These light activities do not have to be long or strenuous. They can signal to the body that it is time to ease into sleep mode. Doing them slowly, with gentle breathing, can bring a sense of calm.

Handling Nighttime Waking

1. **Check for Comfort**
    - If you wake up because you feel too hot, too cold, or in pain, adjust your blankets or sleeping position.
    - Some people find relief with a small, firm pillow between their knees if they lie on their side, helping align the hips and lower back.
2. **Avoid Clock-Watching**
    - Staring at the clock and calculating how many hours of sleep you have left can create stress.
    - If possible, turn the clock's face away or cover it. This helps you avoid the frustration of seeing the minutes tick by.
3. **Limit Long Stretches of Lying Awake**
    - If you cannot fall back to sleep within about 15 or 20 minutes, consider getting up and doing something quiet in dim light, like reading a gentle story or doing a simple puzzle.
    - Once you feel drowsy again, return to bed. Lying awake for too long in bed might cause you to associate the bed with restlessness.
4. **Sip Water, Not Snacks**
    - If you feel thirsty, a small sip of water can help. Try not to drink large amounts so you do not need the bathroom again soon.
    - Avoid sugary or caffeinated drinks, as they could raise energy levels or irritate the bladder.
5. **Calm the Mind**
    - If you wake up worrying, write down concerns on a piece of paper to address the next day. This can keep your thoughts from spinning in circles.
    - Alternatively, do quiet breathing or recall a simple, pleasant scene in your mind, such as a peaceful beach or garden.

Using Naps Wisely

1. **Short Naps**
   - A small rest during the day, like 15 to 30 minutes, can refresh you without messing up nighttime sleep.
   - Longer naps might push your bedtime later or result in tossing and turning at night.
2. **Pick Early Times**
   - If you nap too close to evening, your body might not be ready for bed when night arrives.
   - Early afternoon is often a sweet spot for a quick nap, especially if you had an early morning.
3. **Light Environment**
   - A short doze in a chair near a window with gentle daylight can signal your brain that this is a brief rest, not a full night's sleep.
   - Keep the environment comfortable but not pitch-dark.
4. **Stand Up and Move After**
   - Once your nap time is over, stand up, take a few steps, or stretch. This helps the body transition back to alertness.
   - Drinking a small glass of water or washing your face can also help you feel fully awake.

Naps can be helpful, but if you find they lead to nighttime insomnia, consider skipping them or making them shorter.

Natural Aids to Consider

1. **Herbal Teas**
   - Chamomile or a mild blend of herbs like lavender or lemon balm can be soothing.
   - Drink them an hour before bed, so you have time to use the bathroom before sleep.
2. **Essential Oils**
   - Some people find the scent of lavender or other gentle fragrances relaxing. A few drops on a pillow or in a diffuser might ease tension.
   - Be sure the scent is not overpowering, and check for allergies or sensitivities.

3. **Warm Milk**
    - This classic idea might help some individuals. Warm milk contains a small amount of tryptophan, which the body can use to make calming chemicals.
    - However, if dairy upsets your digestion, try a different mild beverage.
4. **Light Snacks**
    - If you are a bit hungry, a small, balanced snack (like half a banana with a spoonful of peanut butter) might keep hunger from disturbing sleep.
    - Avoid sweets or heavy meals that could unsettle the stomach.
5. **Over-the-Counter Sleep Helpers**
    - Some people use mild sleep aids like melatonin. This hormone can help guide the body's internal clock, but it is not a magic fix for everyone.
    - Always talk to a doctor or pharmacist about potential interactions or correct dosages, especially if you take other medications.

Common Sleep Disorders to Know

Sometimes, poor sleep can be a sign of a specific condition:

1. **Insomnia**
    - This refers to having trouble falling asleep or staying asleep, even when you have time to rest.
    - Chronic insomnia lasts for at least a few nights each week over a month or more.
2. **Sleep Apnea**
    - A disorder where breathing stops briefly during sleep, causing loud snoring or gasps for air.
    - Untreated sleep apnea can lead to daytime tiredness and raise risks for other health issues.
3. **Restless Legs Syndrome (RLS)**
    - An urge to move the legs, often with odd feelings like tingling or crawling, mainly when lying down.
    - RLS can disrupt falling asleep and lead to frequent awakenings.
4. **Periodic Limb Movement Disorder**

- Different from RLS, it involves involuntary leg or arm twitches during the night that might disturb rest.
5. **Circadian Rhythm Disorders**
    - The body clock might be out of sync with normal sleep times, making it tough to fall asleep or wake up at desired hours.

If you suspect a sleep disorder, it can help to talk with a healthcare professional. Some tests, like a sleep study, might show what is happening during the night.

Avoiding Too Many Sleep Medications

Prescription sleep medications might help for short-term issues, but there can be risks:

1. **Dependency**
    - Some drugs lead to reliance, meaning the body struggles to sleep without them.
    - Stopping these medications can cause rebound insomnia, making sleep worse.
2. **Side Effects**
    - Some people feel groggy or dizzy the next day, which can raise the risk of falls.
    - Others experience confusion or poor memory if the drug remains in their system.
3. **Tolerance**
    - Over time, the body might get used to a certain dosage, leading to less effect and a need for higher amounts.
    - This can create a cycle of increasing medication use, which might not be safe for older adults.

If you do use prescription sleep meds, follow the guidelines carefully and check in with your doctor regularly to discuss any changes in your sleep or side effects.

Tracking Sleep to Identify Patterns

1. **Use a Sleep Diary**
    - Write down bedtime, approximate time you fall asleep, nighttime awakenings, final wake time, and how rested you feel in the morning.

- Note factors like caffeine intake, exercise, or stressful events to see if there is a pattern.
  2. **Apps and Devices**
     - Some people use wearable gadgets or phone apps to monitor sleep duration and quality.
     - While they are not always accurate, they can show general trends, such as how often you wake up.
  3. **Look for Clear Links**
     - Does a certain snack or late caffeine keep you up?
     - Do you sleep better after mild walks or on days with fresh air? Identifying these links can guide positive changes.

Social and Environmental Factors

1. **Bed Partner**
   - If you share a bed with someone who snores loudly or tosses and turns, it might affect your rest.
   - Using separate blankets or, in some cases, sleeping in different beds can help if both partners agree it is best for a good night's sleep.
2. **Noise in the Neighborhood**
   - Busy streets or neighbors might create late-night sounds.
   - White noise machines or earplugs can help, or you might speak politely with neighbors if their noise is consistent and disturbing.
3. **Evening Activities**
   - Chatting with friends or playing quiet games can be pleasant, but avoid intense arguments or emotional TV shows close to bedtime.
   - Keep the mood calm as night approaches.

Tips for Waking Up More Refreshed

1. **Gentle Morning Light**
   - Opening curtains soon after waking can help reset your internal clock, telling the brain that it is daytime.
   - Natural light can also lift mood and energy levels.
2. **Stretch in Bed**

- Flex your feet, roll your wrists, and gently arch your back before standing up. This can warm up stiff muscles.
- A calm start helps you avoid rushing, which can strain the body.
3. **Sip Water**
    - Overnight, the body can lose fluids. A glass of water in the morning can help you feel more awake.
    - If you enjoy a warm drink like tea, that can also be soothing, but remember to watch out for caffeine intake if it affects your sleep later.
4. **Plan a Pleasant Activity**
    - Having a small positive focus in the morning—like reading a short uplifting article or working on a simple puzzle—can make the waking process more enjoyable.
    - This helps you avoid feeling grumpy or rushed.
5. **Stand or Move**
    - If you feel stiffness, take a short walk around the house or step outside for fresh air if possible.
    - Light movement can reduce morning sluggishness and signal to the body that the new day has begun.

When to Seek Advice

If you have tried these tips and still struggle with poor sleep or ongoing tiredness, it may be time to talk with a doctor or a sleep specialist. Here are signs that professional input might help:

- You are often awake for long stretches at night and feel too tired to do your normal tasks the next day.
- You or your partner notices gasping or pauses in breathing while you sleep, suggesting possible sleep apnea.
- You experience frequent tingling or restless feelings in your legs at night.
- You find that none of your changes seem to help, and you are feeling more worried or sad about sleeping.

A healthcare professional can check whether an underlying condition is at play or if a specific medication is disrupting your rest. They can also guide you toward advanced treatments or therapies that match your health needs.

CHAPTER 12: BUILDING STRONG SOCIAL TIES

Having supportive relationships is important for people of every age, but it can be especially helpful for older adults. Spending time with others can lift spirits, provide help when needed, and keep the mind active. Over the years, social circles might shift due to retirement, moves, or changing family situations. Still, staying connected is worth the effort. In this chapter, we will look at unique ways older adults can form or strengthen social ties without repeating details from earlier discussions. We will also include ideas for friendships, family connections, community activities, and social technology, all in simple terms that a child could understand.

Why Social Connections Matter for Older Adults

1. **Emotional Health**
   - Spending time with people who care about you can ease feelings of loneliness or sadness.
   - A friendly voice on the phone or a familiar face around you can give a sense of comfort and belonging.
2. **Mental Stimulation**
   - Chats, card games, or group hobbies help keep the brain active.
   - When you share stories or ask questions, the mind stays engaged, which can support clearer thinking.
3. **Physical Well-Being**
   - Friends and family might encourage you to go on walks, attend gentle fitness classes, or try new healthy habits together.
   - Having a buddy for daily movement can make activities more enjoyable and reduce the chance you will skip them.
4. **Practical Assistance**
   - A neighbor might help carry groceries if you need a hand. A friend might drive you to an appointment. Family members may help with chores.
   - People who have a strong network often find it easier to manage unexpected problems.
5. **Shared Joy and Comfort**
   - Good news or personal achievements feel sweeter when shared with trusted individuals.

- If you go through a hard time, having people to talk to can reduce stress.

Social ties do not have to be huge groups or loud gatherings. Even a small circle of close relationships can bring these benefits.

Overcoming Barriers to Social Connections

1. **Transportation**
    - If driving has become difficult, find out about local bus services, volunteer driving groups, or rides from friends.
    - Some places have senior transportation programs that pick you up for community events or doctor visits.
2. **Energy Levels**
    - Medical conditions might make it tough to go out. Consider short visits or simpler outings that match your energy.
    - Invite people over for low-key gatherings where you can rest if needed.
3. **Hearing or Vision Concerns**
    - If hearing loss makes group settings hard, look for quieter spots with minimal background noise.
    - For vision problems, choose well-lit areas and ask for large-print materials if you are attending an event.
4. **Anxiety**
    - Feeling nervous about meeting new people or going to new places is common, especially if it has been a while.
    - Start with small steps, like a short phone call or an online group chat. Gradually work up to in-person visits.
5. **Location Changes**
    - Moving to a new home or retirement community can separate you from old friends, but it can also open chances to make new acquaintances.
    - Seek local activity boards or news bulletins to discover clubs or events in your area.

Finding New Friendships

1. **Senior Centers**
    - Many towns have centers where older adults can join group exercise classes, art sessions, or card games.
    - It is a chance to meet people with similar life experiences.
2. **Hobby Groups**
    - If you enjoy knitting, chess, or gardening, look for clubs that focus on these activities.
    - Sharing a pastime helps start conversations naturally.
3. **Volunteering**
    - Helping at a library, an animal shelter, or a food pantry can connect you with others who have caring hearts.
    - Volunteering not only benefits others but also brings a sense of purpose.
4. **Places of Worship**
    - Religious communities often hold social gatherings and group meals.
    - They might organize small study groups or charity events where you can build closer friendships.
5. **Online Groups**
    - If traveling is hard, online forums or social media groups can link you with people who share your interests.
    - Focus on smaller or age-friendly groups to avoid feeling lost in a large online crowd.

Staying Close with Family

1. **Plan Regular Calls**
    - Set a consistent day or time each week to catch up with adult children or grandkids.
    - A short check-in might be enough to feel connected, even if you live far apart.
2. **Use Video Chats**
    - Video calls let you see faces, which can be more personal than a regular phone call.
    - Ask a tech-savvy friend, relative, or local library helper to show you how to set up a simple video chat on a tablet or phone.

3. **Share Photos and Stories**
    - If you have old family photos, consider labeling them with dates or funny memories to pass on.
    - Younger relatives might enjoy hearing stories about what life was like before computers or cell phones were common.
4. **Involve Younger Generations**
    - Grandchildren can visit and help with small tasks like setting up a smartphone or playing a board game.
    - Teaching them a skill you have (like sewing or simple cooking) can strengthen bonds across ages.
5. **Plan Occasional Gatherings**
    - Birthdays or low-key meals can bring the family together.
    - If distance is an issue, consider rotating who hosts, or plan a get-together once or twice a year at a midpoint location.

Ideas for Group Activities

1. **Book Clubs**
    - Reading a simple book and chatting about it can be fun. Book clubs often meet monthly, giving everyone time to finish reading at their own pace.
    - If reading an entire book feels too heavy, try a short story club or ask participants to share any article or poem they like.
2. **Movie Nights**
    - Invite a few friends to watch a classic or a new release at your home. Pause occasionally if someone needs a break.
    - Sharing popcorn and discussing the film afterward can lead to lively chats.
3. **Craft Circles**
    - Gather for artsy projects like scrapbooking, painting, or making holiday cards.
    - Everyone can bring their own supplies, and you share tips or designs. Even beginners can have a good time trying something new.
4. **Outdoor Walks**
    - If mobility allows, strolling in a park or around the block with one or two people can be both social and healthy.

- Pick paths that are not too steep. Bring water and maybe a small snack.
5. **Friendly Contests**
    - Lighthearted competitions like dominoes, trivia quizzes, or board games can add excitement.
    - Keep the atmosphere fun, not intense, so everyone can enjoy without pressure.

Building Connections Online

1. **Social Media Basics**
    - Platforms like Facebook or others can help you reconnect with distant friends or relatives.
    - Watch privacy settings carefully and accept friend requests only from people you know or trust.
2. **Video Group Chats**
    - Some services let multiple people join the same video call. This can be like a virtual party, where each person is at home but can see and talk to everyone.
    - Plan a time that works for all. Maybe show a pet or a new craft project while chatting.
3. **Online Learning**
    - Some websites offer free courses on topics like history, foreign languages, or computer basics.
    - Many classes include discussion forums where you can post messages and talk with classmates from around the world.
4. **Email Exchanges**
    - Sending letters through email can be a modern version of pen pals.
    - Write short updates about your day, include photos if you like, and encourage the other person to reply in their own time.
5. **Safety Tips**
    - Never share personal details (address, bank info, social security number) with people you meet online.
    - If someone's messages make you uncomfortable, stop interacting and block or report them if needed.

Maintaining Friendships

1. **Reach Out Regularly**
   - A quick text or short call to say "I'm thinking of you" can show you care.
   - Simple gestures, like remembering a friend's birthday or sending a seasonal card, help keep ties strong.
2. **Offer Help**
   - If you learn a friend is sick, see if they need a ride to the clinic or a small grocery run. If you are not able to drive yourself, you might organize support by calling shared friends or setting up a delivery.
3. **Be Open About Needs**
   - If you have trouble hearing and prefer a quiet cafe, let your friend know. Good friends will often be glad to meet in a spot that suits you.
   - If finances are tight, look for free or low-cost activities, like a walk in the park or a home-based tea chat.
4. **Balance Giving and Receiving**
   - Healthy friendships involve both sides giving time, care, or support. It is okay to ask for small favors, but also look for ways you can help your friend in return.
   - Being mindful that each person has limits can keep the friendship strong and respectful.
5. **Respect Differences**
   - Friends may not share every opinion. That is okay. Listen politely, and if a topic causes heated disagreement, switch to a kinder subject.
   - Staying open-minded can keep friendships from breaking over small disputes.

Local Community Involvement

1. **Library Events**
   - Libraries often host talks, art shows, or clubs for older adults.
   - You might discover new interests or connect with people who visit the same library branch.
2. **Town Gatherings**

- Some neighborhoods or towns hold fairs, music nights, or potluck dinners.
- Taking part in these events can lead to casual conversations that spark new acquaintances.

3. **Charity and Service Clubs**
   - Groups like the Lions Club or Rotary Club are community service organizations that welcome older adults.
   - You can support local causes while meeting folks who share a wish to be helpful.

4. **Local Sports or Walking Teams**
   - Some areas have walking clubs or low-intensity sports groups where seniors can team up.
   - This might add a sense of camaraderie and fun while staying active.

5. **Workshops and Classes**
   - Community education programs might offer short lessons in cooking, painting, or basic computer use.
   - Learning side by side can help break the ice with new people.

Helping Others for Deeper Bonds

1. **Mentoring Younger People**
   - If you have skills like woodworking, gardening, or sewing, sharing that knowledge can be a rewarding way to connect with younger folks.
   - Mentoring can happen through local youth centers or church groups.

2. **Local Schools**
   - Some schools welcome seniors to read with children, help in the library, or assist with simple tasks.
   - This can be a fun way to stay active in the community and help the next generation.

3. **Letter Writing to Service Members**
   - Some organizations link older adults with soldiers or others who are away from home for long periods.
   - Sending letters or care packages can create meaningful connections, even if you never meet in person.

4. **Shared Gardening**

- If you enjoy plants, see if there is a community garden. You can grow vegetables or flowers with a group, then share advice or harvest.
- Working side by side often encourages friendly chats and teamwork.

5. **Donation Drives**
    - Whether it is collecting canned goods for a food bank or gently used clothes for a shelter, group efforts can bring people together around a good cause.
    - You get to meet like-minded folks who want to make a difference.

Keeping Yourself Open to New Bonds

1. **Positive Attitude**
    - If you assume you will not get along with anyone, that negative thought can block new friendships.
    - Reminding yourself that most people appreciate kindness can help you stay open to chatting with strangers who might become friends.
2. **Willingness to Listen**
    - Show genuine interest in others' stories or challenges. Listening more than talking at first can make people feel valued and can open doors to closer connections.
    - Ask simple follow-up questions without prying into personal details.
3. **Adapt to Modern Ways**
    - Technology might feel daunting, but learning basic tools like texting or video calling can expand your options for staying in touch.
    - If using a computer is new to you, start small with an email account or a simplified device designed for older adults.
4. **Acknowledge Past Losses**
    - If you have lost close friends or a partner, you might worry about forming new relationships. While it is normal to grieve, allowing new people into your life can bring fresh warmth.
    - It does not mean forgetting those you cared about; it is simply adding to your circle.
5. **Patience and Persistence**

- Real friendships often form over time. If one group or event does not feel right, try another.
- Keep looking for places where you feel comfortable. Sometimes it only takes one good connection to improve social life.

Combating Loneliness at Home

Even with efforts to get out, there might be times you are mostly home-based:

1. **Set Small Daily Goals**
   - Call a different friend on each day of the week, or send a short note to someone online.
   - This spreads out contact and gives you something to look forward to.
2. **Use the Radio or Audiobooks**
   - Having friendly voices or stories in the background can ease the hush in the house.
   - But balance it with actual human connection whenever possible.
3. **Try a Pet**
   - A pet like a cat or a small dog can provide companionship. Caring for them adds structure to the day.
   - If you cannot have a pet full-time, consider offering to watch a friend's pet occasionally or volunteering at an animal shelter for short visits.
4. **Display Photos**
   - Placing pictures of family, friends, or past events around your home can remind you of your social ties and happy memories.
   - Rotate them now and then, or add new ones if you get them.
5. **Phone Trees or Buddy Systems**
   - Some communities have phone tree programs where participants call each other at set times, making sure everyone is doing okay.
   - A buddy system pairs you with a neighbor or friend so you can check in daily or weekly. It can be reassuring to know someone will notice if you need help.

Balancing Alone Time and Social Time

While strong connections are crucial, everyone needs a balance:

1. **Notice Your Preferences**
   - Some people love daily gatherings; others prefer smaller, less frequent interactions.
   - It is okay to manage your social calendar so it fits your comfort level.
2. **Take Breaks**
   - If you get tired easily, limit how long you spend at group events. Leave when you start to feel worn out, rather than pushing yourself to stay.
   - Friends should understand if you need shorter visits.
3. **Enjoy Personal Hobbies**
   - Having quiet hobbies like reading, solving puzzles, or listening to music can refresh you before your next social meeting.
   - A balanced lifestyle mixes these peaceful periods with time spent around others.
4. **Communicate Boundaries**
   - Let family or friends know if certain visiting times are not good for you (for instance, if you nap in the afternoon).
   - Doing so can prevent misunderstandings or stress.
5. **Stay True to Yourself**
   - You do not have to say yes to every invitation. Only go to activities that make you feel good.
   - Quality of contact is often more important than quantity.

CHAPTER 13: AVOIDING HARMFUL HABITS

All of us have daily routines. Some habits make our lives better—like brushing our teeth or tidying up our homes. Other habits might be harmful to our health. Harmful habits can come in many forms: smoking, using too much alcohol, sitting too long, or even letting negative thoughts shape how we act. As the years go by, these harmful habits can weigh on the body and mind, causing problems that might be avoided with awareness and small changes.

In this chapter, we will look at why harmful habits appear, how they affect older adults in particular, and what can be done to address them. We will not repeat the points covered in earlier chapters about nutrition, daily movement, or stress. Instead, we will focus on issues like smoking, heavy drinking, drug misuse, and a few other risky choices that can sneak into everyday life. We will also share positive steps for breaking free from these habits and replacing them with safer options that help protect health and comfort.

Why Harmful Habits Take Hold

1. **Past Influences**
    - Often, habits start early in life. Someone might pick up smoking in their teens, never knowing how hard it can be to stop later on.
    - If those around us also smoke or drink a lot, it can feel normal. Over time, it becomes a routine that is tricky to end.
2. **Relief or Escape**
    - Some older adults use harmful habits to seek relief from aches or sadness. They might turn to a drink to numb pain or smoke a cigarette to calm nerves.
    - Even though these actions may bring short-term comfort, they can harm the body over time.
3. **Lack of Support**
    - Breaking a habit can be hard without encouragement from friends or family. If someone lives alone or feels they have no one to lean on, they might keep the habit.
    - In other cases, people might not realize the extent of the damage a habit is causing until problems appear.
4. **Feelings of Hopelessness**
    - A harmful habit might take root if a person believes nothing else can help them cope with daily problems.

- Changing a longtime routine can seem impossible, so they give up on trying.

Harmful habits are not a sign of weakness or bad character. They usually start for understandable reasons. But if left unchecked, they can harm many parts of life—body, mood, finances, and relationships. The good news is that it is rarely too late to change.

Smoking and Tobacco Use

1. **How Smoking Affects Health**
    - Smoking can harm the lungs and heart, raise blood pressure, and lessen oxygen flow. It might lead to breathing difficulties, coughing, and a higher risk of serious conditions.
    - Tobacco smoke contains chemicals that damage cells. This makes healing slower and can raise the chance of getting certain illnesses.
2. **Why It Can Be Hard to Stop**
    - Tobacco contains nicotine, which can create strong cravings. It can feel like the body depends on nicotine to feel "normal."
    - For many, smoking also becomes tied to daily routines—for instance, having a cigarette with morning coffee or after a meal.
3. **Benefits of Stopping**
    - Even if someone has smoked for decades, stopping can lead to better breathing, a lower chance of new health problems, and more stamina for daily activities.
    - Over time, the body can repair some of the damage. Breathing might become easier, and circulation can improve.
4. **Strategies to Stop**
    - **Talk to a Doctor**: Medical professionals might suggest nicotine patches, gum, or other aids to lessen cravings.
    - **Find Alternatives**: If the urge to hold something arises, some choose sugar-free mints or straws to keep their hands and mouth busy.
    - **Join a Support Group**: Many communities have groups for people who are trying to stop smoking. Sharing stories can bring hope and reduce isolation.
    - **Set Rewards for Progress**: Find a healthy treat or small item to mark the day you go without smoking. These small acknowledgments can help you stick to your plan.

Stopping smoking is not always easy, but it can bring real relief to the body. Shortness of breath might lessen, and the risk of certain illnesses can start to decline. One step at a time is enough to begin.

Heavy Drinking of Alcohol

1. **Why Older Adults Might Drink More**
   - Some people find that in retirement, they have more free time and fewer responsibilities, which might lead them to drink as a pastime.
   - Others might use alcohol to handle sadness, loneliness, or physical pain.
2. **Risks of High Alcohol Use**
   - Drinking too much alcohol can impair balance, raising the risk of falls.
   - It can strain the liver, damage the stomach lining, and affect how medications work.
   - Older adults might feel the effects more strongly because the body processes alcohol more slowly with age.
3. **How to Spot a Problem**
   - If a person feels they need a drink to relax every day, it might signal an unhealthy reliance.
   - Increased tolerance—needing more to feel any effect—can be a warning sign.
   - Poor memory or confusion can be tied to heavy drinking, especially in an older body.
4. **Healthier Ways to Cope**
   - **Limit or Avoid Alcohol**: If you choose to drink, keep it modest. For many older adults, one drink per day or less may be enough.
   - **Find Social Support**: Talk to friends or family about your concerns, or join a group that helps with alcohol issues.
   - **Explore New Pastimes**: If boredom leads to drinking, find other ways to fill time—like crafts, puzzles, or phone chats.
   - **Seek Counseling**: Therapists can help address the deeper reasons for heavy alcohol use and suggest coping strategies.

Cutting back on alcohol, or even removing it entirely, can allow the body to function more smoothly. Blood pressure might improve, and thoughts can become clearer. If quitting outright feels daunting, start by reducing the number of drinks gradually, or ask a healthcare provider for help.

Medication and Drug Misuse

1. **Prescription Medications**
   - Many older adults take prescriptions for conditions like pain or anxiety. These drugs can be helpful if used properly.
   - Problems arise when people take more than prescribed or mix medications without telling their doctor.
2. **Over-the-Counter Drugs**
   - Pain relievers or sleeping aids bought at the store can be harmful if used too often or in high amounts.
   - Some drugs interact with each other, causing side effects like confusion or dizziness.
3. **Misuse or Dependence**
   - Older adults might forget they already took their medicine and accidentally take extra.
   - In some cases, a person might rely on pills to cope with emotional upset, leading to dependence.
4. **Preventing Medication Problems**
   - **Keep a Medication List**: Write down the names and doses of every medicine, including over-the-counter items. Update it when changes occur.
   - **Use a Pill Organizer**: These containers have compartments for each day of the week, helping you track daily doses.
   - **Ask About Interactions**: When starting a new drug, check with a pharmacist about safe combinations.
   - **Avoid Sharing**: A medicine that helps one person might harm another, so never share prescriptions.
5. **Street Drugs and Other Substances**
   - Though less common in older age, misuse of street drugs or untested herbal substances can be risky.
   - These can interfere with prescription medications, and their quality might be uncertain, leading to harmful chemicals in the body.

Using medications in a safe manner can prevent complications like falls, confusion, or even hospitalization. Regular communication with medical professionals is key.

Overeating or Excessive Snacking

1. **When Eating Becomes a Habit**
   - Some people eat out of boredom or when feeling anxious. This can lead to weight gain or stress on the digestive system.
   - If older adults have easy access to snacks and do not move around much, they might slip into overeating.
2. **Risks for Older Adults**
   - Extra weight can strain knees, hips, and feet, making it harder to walk or stay active.
   - Too much sugar or salt might raise blood pressure or disrupt healthy blood sugar levels.
3. **Finding Balance**
   - **Portion Awareness**: Even nutritious foods can become a problem in large amounts. Learning what a healthy portion looks like can help.
   - **Satisfying Activities**: If reaching for snacks is a response to boredom, try a puzzle, phone call, or short stroll instead.
   - **Mindful Eating**: Pay attention while eating. Notice flavors and chew slowly rather than munching mindlessly in front of the TV.
   - **Seek Guidance**: A doctor or nutritionist can suggest ways to manage overeating without feeling deprived.

Excessive snacking might not seem as obviously harmful as smoking or drinking, but it can still lead to gradual health declines. By noticing triggers and building a healthier relationship with food, a person can take a step away from this harmful habit.

Sitting for Long Hours

1. **Why It Happens**
   - Retirement can mean less need to move around. Some older adults have conditions that make walking painful, so they sit in one spot for most of the day.
   - Long TV watching or computer use might become the main pastime.
2. **Risks of Long Sitting**

- The body's joints might become stiff, circulation can slow, and muscles might weaken. This raises the risk of falls and injuries.
- Extended sitting might also affect mood, leading to a feeling of being stuck or bored.

3. **Breaking the Sitting Habit**
    - **Set Timers**: Every 30 or 60 minutes, stand up, do a quick stretch or take a few steps, then return to sitting if needed.
    - **Move in Small Ways**: Even lifting arms or doing gentle leg stretches in a chair can boost blood flow.
    - **Foster New Routines**: If you watch TV, march lightly in place during commercials, or do simple arm movements.
    - **Safe Walking**: When possible, short walks around the block or inside a store can help break up long periods of sitting.

Though not always labeled a harmful habit, excessive sitting can quietly reduce a person's overall health. Keeping the body in motion, even a little, helps maintain flexibility and comfort as time passes.

Negative Self-Talk or Hopeless Thinking

1. **What It Looks Like**
    - Telling oneself, "I cannot do anything right," or "I am too old to try new things."
    - Feeling constant regret about the past and believing the future holds no positive outlook.
2. **Why It Is Harmful**
    - The mind can start believing negative thoughts, reducing energy and interest in activities.
    - It may lead to isolating oneself from friends, giving up on health routines, and ignoring symptoms that should be treated.
3. **Ways to Address It**
    - **Notice Thoughts**: The first step is realizing when negative statements pop up.
    - **Use Gentle Replacements**: If the mind says, "I am useless," replace it with, "I can still learn or help in small ways."
    - **Practice Gratitude**: A short list of daily positives can remind you of what is still good, such as a safe home or a caring friend.
    - **Consider Counseling**: A counselor or therapist can guide older adults in shifting their mindset to more balanced thoughts.

Negative self-talk might not seem like a physical habit, yet it can shape behavior in harmful ways. By gently steering thoughts toward hope or acceptance, a person can open up opportunities for more fulfilling experiences.

Breaking Free: Steps to Overcome Harmful Habits

1. **Awareness**
    - The first key is to admit a certain behavior might be causing harm. Without recognizing the problem, it is hard to take the next step.
    - Writing down each time you engage in the harmful habit—be it drinking, smoking, or overeating—can highlight patterns.
2. **Set Clear Goals**
    - Be specific, like "I will reduce smoking from 10 cigarettes a day to 5 by next month," or "I will only have 1 alcoholic drink at social events."
    - Goals work best if they are realistic, measurable, and not overly strict, so you do not feel defeated.
3. **Seek Guidance**
    - **Medical Experts**: Doctors, pharmacists, or addiction specialists can offer tools to quit or cut back.
    - **Support Circles**: Whether a formal group or a few friends who keep each other accountable, moral support makes a big difference.
    - **Online Resources**: Some websites or hotlines provide tips for stopping harmful habits. Be sure to trust reliable sources.
4. **Replace Harmful Habits**
    - Simply stopping a habit can leave an empty space. Fill it with a healthy action: go for a short walk instead of lighting a cigarette, call a friend instead of opening a drink, or prepare a cup of herbal tea when snack urges strike.
    - Replacement keeps the mind and body busy, reducing the craving to go back to old patterns.
5. **Reward Progress**
    - Small positive acknowledgments can be encouraging. An older adult might put money saved from not buying cigarettes into a jar for a fun treat, like a nice dinner or new slippers.
    - Tracking how many days you have stayed within a goal also helps sustain motivation.

6. **Plan for Slips**
    - People often slip back into harmful habits now and then, especially when stressed.
    - A slip does not mean failure; it is a chance to learn. Look at what caused the slip and adjust strategies to handle it better next time.

Handling Social Pressure

1. **Friends or Family Who Use the Same Habit**
    - If others around you also smoke or drink heavily, they might feel uneasy if you try to stop, worrying about changes in the relationship.
    - Let them know why you are making changes. Invite them to join you, but if they are not ready, set boundaries about when or where you will meet.
2. **Polite Declines**
    - Practice calm ways to say "No, thank you," if someone offers you a cigarette or a second drink. It does not have to be rude; just be firm.
    - If you worry about hurting feelings, you can say something like, "I am cutting back for my health."
3. **Choosing Safe Spaces**
    - If going to a bar is too tempting, suggest meeting in a coffee shop or a friend's home where there will not be pressure to drink.
    - If a family member smokes indoors, arrange visits in a spot with fresh air or open windows.
4. **Reassessing Certain Friendships**
    - In some cases, a person might realize that certain friends only ever meet up to smoke or drink. If that is the main connection, it might be time to find new social outlets.
    - This does not mean cutting ties completely, but limiting time spent in settings that undo your progress might help.

Mental and Emotional Support

1. **Therapy or Counseling**

- Talking to a professional can uncover the deeper feelings that lead to harmful habits.
- Therapists can teach coping skills for stress, sadness, or worry that do not rely on unhealthy behaviors.

2. **Mindful Techniques**
    - Techniques like slow breathing or short visualization can calm the urge to do something harmful.
    - For instance, if you feel a craving to smoke, sit quietly, close your eyes, and breathe in and out slowly until the craving passes.

3. **Medical Check-Ins**
    - Regular doctor visits can track progress—like breathing improvements or healthier blood pressure—and remind you why the change is worth it.
    - Blood tests or screenings might show how your body is healing over time.

4. **Family and Friends**
    - Share your progress with loved ones who are supportive. They might cheer you on or help you steer clear of triggers.
    - Leaning on close people can lessen loneliness that often leads to unhealthy behaviors.

Benefits of Removing Harmful Habits

1. **Physical Relief**
    - Stopping smoking can boost lung capacity, making it easier to walk or climb steps.
    - Cutting back on alcohol might lead to clearer thinking, steadier balance, and fewer trips to the bathroom at night.

2. **Emotional Gains**
    - Overcoming a habit can bring a sense of control and confidence, replacing feelings of shame or guilt.
    - Better sleep or calmer moods may follow once certain substances are reduced or stopped.

3. **Financial Savings**
    - Cigarettes, alcohol, or even frequent snack runs can be costly. Money saved can go toward new hobbies, helpful devices, or maybe a modest outing.
    - The pressure of not having enough funds for other needs might lessen.

4. **Improved Relationships**
   - Friends and family may be relieved to see you healthier.
   - You might enjoy social events more without worrying about your habit interfering.
5. **Stronger Independence**
   - Harmful habits can make a person feel trapped. Moving past them can lead to a greater sense of freedom.
   - Being able to rely on your own choices rather than a harmful routine might preserve independence in older age.

Replacing Harmful Patterns with Positive Ones

1. **Explore New Activities**
   - Trying gentle dance, painting, or cooking simple meals might fill time once given to a harmful habit.
   - Activities can be enjoyable and offer a way to connect with others who share these interests.
2. **Stay Connected**
   - Keep in touch with friends who support your better habits.
   - Join local or online groups for older adults focusing on safer lifestyle choices—like walking clubs or community games.
3. **Check In with Yourself**
   - Ask each day, "How am I feeling? Is anything making me want to fall back on old ways?"
   - Small daily check-ins can catch early warnings before they grow.
4. **Keep Learning**
   - Reading about success stories, health facts, or new coping methods can renew your drive to stay on track.
   - If you use a phone or computer, you might follow trusted resources or sign up for short tips that help you avoid pitfalls.
5. **Give Yourself Time**
   - Changes do not happen overnight. If you spent years smoking or relying on heavy drinks, your mind and body need patience.
   - Each day without the harmful habit is progress, even if it feels slow.

CHAPTER 14: KEEPING THE MIND ACTIVE AND SHARP

The mind is always at work, even when we are not actively thinking about it. It helps us understand daily happenings, remember what matters, and figure out new tasks. As people get older, the brain can change in ways that affect focus and learning, but that does not mean the mind must stop growing. We can continue to keep our thoughts clear and active through simple actions that prompt the brain to stay engaged.

In earlier chapters, we touched on stress, memory, and social connections. In this chapter, we will focus on fresh ideas for keeping the mind active and sharp. We will discuss new topics such as creative thinking, lifelong learning, and ways to challenge the brain without repeating guidance already shared about stress or socializing. By adding more variety to daily thinking, older adults can strengthen mental alertness, feel more motivated, and find extra interest in each day.

Why Keep the Mind Engaged?

1. **Better Daily Function**
    - A sharper mind can handle tasks like following recipes, paying bills, or planning outings with greater ease.
    - It can be simpler to adapt to little changes in the schedule or remember items at the store.
2. **Sense of Purpose**
    - Learning fresh topics or working on a small project can bring a feeling of achievement.
    - Being curious about the world can help older adults feel motivated when they wake up in the morning.
3. **Reduced Risk of Mental Slowdown**
    - While aging naturally shifts brain function, mental exercises may slow certain kinds of decline or keep the mind alert for longer.
    - The brain can form new connections at any age if it is used and challenged in healthy ways.
4. **Emotional Uplift**
    - Finding pleasure in thinking, pondering, or creating can brighten a person's mood.
    - Solving puzzles or learning a new trick can spark positive feelings and reduce boredom.

Keeping the mind active does not require complex math or deep reading if those are not enjoyable. Even simple daily actions, as we will see, can support a clear and responsive brain.

Creative Thinking and Imagination

1. **Artistic Exploration**
   - Drawing or coloring: Even basic doodles can relax the mind while inviting new ideas. Using colored pencils or markers on simple designs can be soothing.
   - Clay or dough: Shaping something with hands can lead to a sense of accomplishment and strengthen fine motor skills.
   - Music making: Trying a basic instrument, like a small keyboard or a simple drum, can stimulate the parts of the brain linked to rhythm and pattern.
2. **Creative Writing**
   - Journaling: Write a few sentences about daily observations or thoughts. This can sharpen recall and help process ideas.
   - Poetry: Short, playful poems can capture small moments or feelings without needing fancy words.
   - Small stories: If you have a vivid memory, turning it into a short story can be both fun and mentally stimulating.
3. **Craft Projects**
   - Easy crafts with paper, fabric, or yarn can challenge the brain to plan and create.
   - Even an older adult with limited hand strength might enjoy simple tasks like gluing decorations onto a card or folding paper shapes.
4. **Mindful Observations**
   - Walk around the yard or a safe space, noticing tiny details like colors of leaves or shapes of clouds.
   - Draw or describe what you see in a simple notebook. This encourages the mind to focus on the present and record details.

Creative thinking is not about being perfect or producing a masterpiece. It is about inviting the brain to see or do something new, which can sharpen attention and spark fresh ideas.

Lifelong Learning Opportunities

1. **Library Classes**
   - Some libraries offer workshops, talks, or basic lessons in topics like local history or basic computer use.
   - Signing up for a simple class can open the door to meeting others and learning new facts.
2. **Online Lessons**
   - Free websites or video channels teach subjects like a new language, how to fix things around the house, or how to use a smartphone better.
   - Many older adults find enjoyment in short tutorials that they can pause and replay as needed.
3. **Personal Tutoring**
   - A neighbor, grandchild, or volunteer might offer to share knowledge on a subject you want to explore, like baking bread or using email.
   - Learning face-to-face can provide a more personal feel, and you can ask questions right away.
4. **Safe Practice**
   - If you are nervous about technology, start small, like sending an email to one friend or using a simple app on a phone.
   - Over time, confidence grows, and you might try more advanced tasks, such as editing pictures or joining an online class.

Staying curious is the main idea. Whether it is history, gardening tips, or a brand-new language, each bit of learning helps keep the brain's gears turning.

Simple Brain Challenges at Home

1. **Word and Number Puzzles**
   - Crossword puzzles let you recall words you already know and pick up new ones in a playful way.
   - Sudoku or other number puzzles allow the mind to handle logic without heavy reading.
   - Word scrambles, letter searches, or simple math teasers can also exercise thinking skills.
2. **Memory Games**

- Try placing several small objects on a tray, look at them for a moment, then cover them. Try to recall as many as possible.
- Ask someone to read a list of words, then see how many you can remember in one minute.

3. **Building or Stacking**
    - Stacking blocks or small items can be surprisingly engaging. The brain must plan the balance and shape of each piece.
    - Simple building kits with large pieces can also be fun if eyesight or grip strength is limited.
4. **Guessing Riddles**
    - A friend or family member can pose a riddle like, "I am round and used in cooking. I can be red or green. What am I?" (an apple or a pepper, depending on the clue).
    - Even silly riddles make you think in creative ways, stretching the mind a bit.

These brain challenges do not have to be long. A few minutes here and there may be enough to help the brain feel invigorated.

Mixing Routine with Variety

1. **Shaking Up the Schedule**
    - If you have the same pattern each day—breakfast at the same spot, reading the same newspaper—try small changes.
    - Sit in a different chair, change the order of your tasks, or pick a new route for a daily stroll. The brain adapts to novelty.
2. **Different Types of Activities**
    - Combine mental tasks (like puzzles) with mild movement (like a few steps around the house). This can improve blood flow to the brain.
    - If you usually watch the same TV shows, consider a documentary on a new topic or a show in a different language with subtitles.
3. **Alternate Quiet and Active Tasks**
    - The brain can get tired if it is focused for too long. Rotate between quiet thinking tasks and active tasks like light cleaning or gentle stretching.
    - This variety helps the mind reset and get fresh energy for the next mental challenge.

4. **Try New Foods or Flavors**
    - Tasting different fruits or herbs can engage the senses in unexpected ways.
    - Cooking a simple recipe from a culture you are not used to can spark mental interest in new ingredients.

Small differences in the daily rhythm wake up the brain. It keeps routines from getting dull and encourages continued learning.

Part-Time or Volunteer Work for Mental Stimulation

1. **Finding the Right Fit**
    - Some older adults enjoy a few hours a week at a local shop, library, or community garden.
    - The goal is not to push oneself too hard, but to pick an activity that feels manageable and rewarding.
2. **Benefits of Work or Service**
    - Problem-solving, meeting people, or organizing items are all ways to keep the mind engaged.
    - It also gives a reason to stay active, dress for an outing, and think about new duties.
3. **Being Clear About Limits**
    - If you have health concerns, let the workplace or volunteer coordinator know. They might have tasks that involve sitting or shorter shifts.
    - Be honest about how much time you can give. Even a small schedule can do wonders for mental energy.
4. **Keeping Up with Changes**
    - Part-time roles can teach new skills, like using a modern cash register or storing data on a computer. This continuous learning keeps thoughts sharp.
    - Supervisors or coworkers might share the latest technology or tips, adding fresh knowledge to your day.

A small job or volunteer role might not fit everyone, but it can be a satisfying way to stay engaged with the world while helping others.

Gentle Physical Actions That Boost Brain Power

1. **Coordination Moves**
    - Try tapping your head with one hand while rubbing your belly with the other, then switch. This challenges the brain's coordination.
    - Simple dance steps, even while holding onto a chair for balance, can combine music and movement in a mind-body workout.
2. **Handwork**
    - Activities like knitting, crocheting, or even threading beads can link the brain to fine motor movements, honing focus.
    - The pattern of stitches or bead sorting keeps the mind alert to what comes next.
3. **Rhythmic Actions**
    - Clapping or tapping out a pattern: clap twice, tap your thighs three times, then snap once, and repeat.
    - Changing the order or speed requires attention and can be a playful brain challenge.
4. **Chair Aerobics with Counting**
    - If you lift one leg, count up to five, lower it, then lift the other leg for another count. Focus on counting backward sometimes for an extra challenge.
    - This small tweak (counting backward) can add a mental edge to ordinary stretches.

Even modest body movements can support brain health by improving blood circulation, raising oxygen flow, and forcing the mind to stay on task.

Technology Tools for Brain Training

1. **Brain Game Apps**
    - Some apps offer short exercises in memory, attention, or speed tasks. They adjust to your pace, so they are not overwhelming.
    - If you prefer a bigger screen, these apps might be found on tablets or computers.
2. **Online Tutorials**
    - Websites with step-by-step lessons on crafts, photography, or cooking can keep the mind alert.

- Some let you pause and replay sections to learn at your own speed.
3. **Video or Audio Courses**
    - You might join free "massive open online courses" (MOOCs) about basic science or art.
    - If you find reading text on a screen tiring, audio courses or podcasts can be a great alternative.
4. **Tracking Progress**
    - Some programs let you see how much you practiced or what level you reached. Small improvements can feel good and spur you to continue.
    - If technology feels confusing, ask a friend or family member for a short demonstration. They can help set up an account and show how to navigate.

Technology can be a helpful tool, but it is only one option. If you prefer paper puzzles or in-person classes, that works just as well.

Group Brain Activities

1. **Discussion Circles**
    - Form a small group to talk about news stories or short articles. Each person shares a perspective, keeping the mind engaged in listening and thinking.
    - You do not need to argue over tough topics; choose light or interesting themes to keep the talk pleasant.
2. **Team Puzzles**
    - Crossword puzzles or jigsaw puzzles can be done together. One person might spot something another misses.
    - This merges social time with mental challenges.
3. **Community Learning Events**
    - Some senior centers host workshops where participants learn about topics like local wildlife, crafts, or safe driving tips.
    - Asking questions and listening to a speaker can spark new thoughts.
4. **Chorus or Music Groups**
    - Singing in a small group or playing simple instruments like a hand drum can involve memory (song lyrics or patterns) and teamwork.

- You do not need to be a great singer—just enjoy the shared experience.

Working on mental tasks with others can boost motivation, reduce loneliness, and make learning more fun.

Handling Obstacles to a Sharp Mind

1. **Fatigue**
   - If tiredness is an issue, short mental exercises might be better than lengthy sessions.
   - Try a 5-minute puzzle here, a 10-minute art activity there, spaced throughout the day.
2. **Vision or Hearing Limits**
   - Use large-print books or specialized magnifiers for reading tasks.
   - If hearing is low, pick quiet spaces for group talks or use assistive listening devices.
   - Let others know if you need them to speak clearly or face you when talking.
3. **Memory Slips**
   - Keep notes or reminders for important details if you struggle to recall them.
   - Use a small notebook or phone app to store quick facts, such as a new word you learned.
4. **Health Concerns**
   - If pain makes it hard to sit and focus, explore small intervals of mental tasks. Talk to a doctor about ways to manage pain.
   - If a medication causes drowsiness or foggy thinking, ask if an alternative or different timing is possible.

Adjusting these hurdles ensures that mental activities can stay part of a person's life, rather than being overshadowed by discomfort.

Creating a Mind-Health Routine

1. **Morning Mental Boost**

- Maybe do a short puzzle or read an interesting paragraph when you wake up to warm up the mind.
- Just a few minutes can set a positive tone for the day.
2. **Midday Review**
    - During lunch, think about something new you learned, or read a short fact.
    - You could also teach that fact to a friend or family member later, which helps cement it in your memory.
3. **Evening Reflection**
    - Spend a few minutes looking back on your day. Did you notice anything interesting or learn something fresh?
    - Jot down a short note about it, which trains the brain to recall events more clearly.
4. **Weekly Goals**
    - Perhaps choose a new word in another language or a new recipe each week. Challenge yourself to remember or perform it by week's end.
    - Keep goals modest so that you do not feel pressured.

A regular approach to mental activity can make it second nature. Over time, you might see daily tasks become simpler and your mood remain brighter.

Knowing When to Seek Help

1. **Frequent Confusion**
    - If you notice you are often lost in familiar places or mixing up names to the point it affects daily life, it might be time to see a medical professional.
    - Some conditions, like certain types of memory loss, need early evaluation.
2. **Sudden Changes**
    - Sharp drops in thinking skills, personality shifts, or trouble with words that appear quickly could point to something serious, like a stroke or infection.
    - Seek medical advice right away if you spot such major changes.
3. **Feeling Overwhelmed**

- If you become anxious at the thought of trying new things or get upset easily when you cannot recall details, talk to someone you trust.
            - A counselor or doctor can suggest ways to handle these concerns.
    4. **Medical Screenings**
            - Regular health check-ups can rule out underlying issues that might hurt brain function, such as thyroid problems or vitamin shortages.
            - If you notice persistent tiredness or mental fog, let your doctor know so they can investigate.

While normal aging can slow some mental processes, big or quick changes often deserve professional attention.

Success Stories and Small Wins

1. **Steady Improvement**
    - One person might begin with simple crosswords and find they can gradually handle more difficult ones over time.
    - Another might learn to send emails to grandchildren, enjoying the feeling of staying in touch with modern tools.
2. **Reviving Old Skills**
    - Sometimes older adults recall a skill they had long ago, like playing a basic tune on a piano, and revisit it. The sense of rediscovery can be exciting.
    - This can spark memories and keep the mind lively.
3. **Sharing Knowledge**
    - Teaching someone else (a neighbor or grandchild) how to do a puzzle, a craft, or a simple computer function is a way to keep your own mind sharp while helping others.
    - Explaining steps out loud strengthens your understanding too.
4. **Everyday Gains**
    - Even being able to remember an acquaintance's name more easily or recall a phone number after practicing mental exercises can feel rewarding.
    - These small wins remind you that the brain still adapts and grows.

CHAPTER 15: FINANCIAL AND LEGAL BASICS FOR LATER LIFE

Money decisions can shape many parts of life, especially as people grow older. Having enough funds to cover day-to-day costs, plan for medical needs, and manage bigger expenses can lead to peace of mind. On top of that, certain legal steps—like writing a will—can ensure that your wishes are followed and that family members know how to handle important matters if you can no longer speak for yourself. In this chapter, we will talk about basic money topics and legal measures that older adults might want to explore. We will avoid repeating earlier advice on topics like healthy eating or stress. Instead, we will focus on ways to handle money, watch out for fraud, and get key legal papers in order.

Why Financial Planning Matters in Older Age

1. **Stable Daily Life**
   - It is helpful to feel sure that you can pay for housing, groceries, and bills without constant worry.
   - When finances are organized, you can focus on other parts of life, like hobbies, family, or friends.
2. **Medical and Care Needs**
   - As people get older, medical bills might go up. Planning ahead can help cover these costs or long-term care if needed.
   - Some older adults might choose special insurance or save extra money for health-related expenses.
3. **Helping Family**
   - Some individuals wish to leave money or property to their children, grandchildren, or other loved ones.
   - Clear plans can reduce disagreements among relatives and ease the process of passing on belongings.
4. **Freedom to Make Choices**
   - With a secure financial plan, you can decide if you want to keep working part-time, volunteer, travel locally, or help relatives in small ways.
   - Feeling more in control of money matters can bring a sense of calm.

Finances can look different for everyone. Some might have pensions or retirement funds. Others may rely on smaller incomes. The main idea is to know your resources, set basic goals, and take steps to keep money matters stable.

Creating a Simple Budget

1. **List Monthly Income**
   - Write down money you receive each month, such as a pension, Social Security payments, rental income, or part-time earnings.
   - Include any consistent interest or dividend payments, if you have them.
2. **Track Regular Bills**
   - List regular expenses: rent or mortgage, utility bills (like electricity, gas, water), phone or internet, and insurance.
   - Do not forget smaller recurring costs, like monthly subscriptions or streaming services.
3. **Estimate Food and Basics**
   - Grocery bills might vary, but you can look at receipts over a few weeks to find an average monthly amount.
   - Think about personal care items or household supplies, too.
4. **Include Medical Costs**
   - If you pay a premium for health insurance, note that down.
   - Consider medicines or regular doctor visits. It can help to set aside a certain amount if these costs pop up regularly.
5. **Add Miscellaneous Spending**
   - This might include hobbies, social outings, and small gifts for family.
   - Even if these seem minor, they add up, so including them helps keep a realistic picture of spending.
6. **Check the Bottom Line**
   - Subtract total expenses from total income.
   - If your expenses exceed your income, you might need to reduce certain costs or find ways to bring in a bit more money.
   - If there is a surplus, you can decide whether to save, invest, or spend carefully on activities that matter to you.

A budget can be as simple as writing on paper or using a basic computer spreadsheet. The goal is to see your money flow clearly, so you can make adjustments if something does not fit well.

Handling Debt and Loans

1. **Why Debt Matters**
   - Too much debt can reduce monthly cash flow, making it hard to pay for normal needs.
   - High interest rates on credit cards or personal loans can grow over time, creating financial strain.
2. **Check Interest Rates**
   - If you have multiple debts, note the interest rates on each one. Some might be higher and cost more in the long run.
   - Paying down high-interest debts first can sometimes lower the amount of money lost to interest.
3. **Talking to Lenders**
   - If monthly payments are tough, contact creditors or a reputable credit counselor for guidance.
   - Some lenders might allow a modified payment plan if they know your situation.
4. **Avoiding New Unnecessary Debt**
   - Though it might be tempting to open new credit lines for convenience or special offers, think carefully.
   - Aim to keep borrowing small if you are on a fixed income, unless it is for an urgent need like home repairs.
5. **Use Secured vs. Unsecured Debt Carefully**
   - Secured debt (like a home equity loan) puts your house on the line if you cannot pay. Unsecured debt (like most credit cards) does not directly seize assets but can still harm your credit score or lead to legal trouble.
   - Always weigh the risks before taking on any new debt, especially later in life.

Working toward paying off debt or keeping it to a manageable level can free up funds for other priorities, like medical costs, savings, or small pleasures.

Saving and Investing Basics

1. **Emergency Funds**
   - Having a small stash of money for sudden needs—like a car repair or a surprise bill—can prevent going into debt.

- Many experts suggest a few months' worth of expenses, but even a smaller cushion can help.

2. **Types of Savings Accounts**
   - A regular savings account might have a modest interest rate but is easy to access.
   - Some banks offer higher-yield savings or money market accounts that pay more interest if you keep a certain balance.

3. **Certificates of Deposit (CDs)**
   - CDs can provide a set interest rate for a chosen period (like 6 months or 1 year).
   - You usually cannot withdraw money without a fee until the term ends, but this can be good if you do not need immediate access and want a stable return.

4. **Bonds or Bond Funds**
   - Bonds are loans to governments or companies that pay interest over time.
   - Older adults often consider bonds because they can be less volatile than some stocks, though they still carry risks if the issuer faces trouble.

5. **Stocks or Stock Funds**
   - These can bring higher returns but also higher risks. The market can swing up or down.
   - Some older adults keep a small portion of stocks for potential growth while relying more on stable investments for essential expenses.

6. **Retirement Accounts**
   - If you have an IRA (Individual Retirement Account) or a 401(k) from past employment, you might be withdrawing funds in older age.
   - Pay attention to any required distributions, which are amounts you must take out after a certain age to follow tax rules.

Choosing where to place money depends on comfort with risk, how soon the funds will be needed, and personal goals. It can help to talk with a financial advisor who works with older adults, though be sure to pick someone trustworthy with clear fee structures.

Being Aware of Scams and Fraud

1. **Why Scammers Target Older Adults**
   - Some criminals assume seniors might have savings or be less familiar with modern gadgets.
   - Others use fear tactics, claiming a person's bank account was "hacked" or that a relative needs urgent cash.
2. **Common Tricks**
   - **Phone Scams**: A caller might pretend to be from a government agency, like the IRS, demanding immediate payment or personal details.
   - **Email or Text Phishing**: A message may claim to be your bank, telling you to click a link to fix a problem. In reality, it can steal your login info.
   - **Charity Fraud**: Someone might ask for donations for a fake cause, especially after a disaster or emergency.
   - **Grandparent Scam**: A scammer pretends to be a grandchild in trouble, asking for quick money.
3. **Staying Safe**
   - Never give out personal information (bank account, social security number) to someone who contacts you unexpectedly.
   - If in doubt, hang up the phone, close the email, and directly call your bank or the supposed agency using a known, official number.
   - Talk to family or a trusted friend if you are unsure about a request.
   - Resist pressure to act fast. Genuine banks or agencies rarely demand immediate, secret payments.
4. **Reporting Scams**
   - If you suspect you were tricked or see suspicious activity, contact local authorities or a consumer protection group.
   - Telling your bank right away might help freeze or recover some funds if the scammer gained access to your account.

Insurance Considerations

1. **Health Insurance**
   - Many older adults are on government healthcare programs or may have additional policies that cover things like prescription medicines, vision, or dental.

- Reviewing coverage each year can save money and ensure that your plan still fits your needs.

2. **Long-Term Care Insurance**
    - This type of coverage can help pay for services if you need help with daily tasks later. It might fund assisted living or home health aides.
    - Policies often cost less if you buy them before major health problems appear. Check the terms carefully to see what is included.

3. **Life Insurance**
    - Some people keep life insurance to help family members handle final expenses or pay off debts.
    - Premiums might rise with age, so weigh the cost versus the benefit. If children are grown and you have savings, you might not need as much coverage.

4. **Homeowner's or Renter's Insurance**
    - Ensures belongings and property are protected against theft, fire, and certain accidents.
    - If you own a home, see if extra coverage is wise for floods or earthquakes, depending on your area.

5. **Umbrella Policies**
    - These add extra liability coverage on top of home or auto insurance, which can be helpful if you worry about large claims against you.
    - Not everyone needs this, but some older adults find it brings additional peace of mind.

Insurance can be confusing, so reviewing it carefully or asking an agent to walk you through the details can help you avoid paying for unneeded coverage or missing gaps that matter.

Important Legal Documents

1. **Will**
    - This is a written statement of what happens to your belongings after you pass away. You can name an executor (a person in charge of carrying out your wishes) and list who gets which items or funds.

- Without a valid will, state laws might decide how to divide your belongings, which might not match your preferences.
2. **Living Will or Advance Directive**
    - This paper explains what medical treatments you want or do not want if you cannot speak for yourself.
    - For example, you can say if you want to be put on a machine to help with breathing or if you prefer comfort care only.
3. **Power of Attorney (POA)**
    - This grants someone legal power to handle certain matters for you if you cannot do so.
    - A **durable financial POA** focuses on money tasks, like paying bills from your account. A **healthcare POA** allows someone to speak with doctors and make medical decisions for you.
4. **Trusts**
    - A trust can hold your assets (like a house or investments) for easier transfer to loved ones without going through a public court process called probate.
    - Some trusts might also help manage assets if you become unable to handle them. They can be complex and might require a specialized lawyer.
5. **Beneficiary Designations**
    - Certain accounts (like retirement funds or life insurance) let you name a beneficiary who receives the money directly.
    - Check these designations now and then to ensure they match your current wishes (for instance, if a beneficiary has passed away or if you divorced and remarried).

Legal papers can vary by region, so consider talking with an attorney familiar with local rules to ensure everything is correct and up to date. Updating these papers after major life changes—like the passing of a spouse—is also wise.

Estate Planning Without Stress

1. **Start Simple**
    - You do not need to figure out every detail immediately. Begin with a basic will or by naming a trusted person under a POA.
    - Later, you can refine or expand your plans as you learn more.
2. **Keep Loved Ones Informed**

- Let close family or friends know where you store important documents, such as wills or insurance details.
- If you have set up a POA, make sure that person understands your preferences and is willing to act on your behalf.
3. **Review Every Few Years**
    - Laws and personal circumstances change. A will written 10 years ago might no longer reflect your current plans.
    - A quick check might confirm everything is still good or show if changes are needed.
4. **Ask for Guidance**
    - Some senior centers host legal aid sessions where lawyers give free or reduced-fee advice to older adults.
    - If you have complex finances, a specialized estate attorney might help with trusts or tax strategies.

Estate planning should not be scary. It is a method to ensure that what you have goes where you want it to go and that your medical wishes are honored if you cannot speak for yourself.

Protecting Documents

1. **Safe Storage**
    - Put wills, POA forms, insurance policies, and property papers in a secure place, like a fire-resistant box or a safe deposit box at the bank.
    - Keep copies in a separate location to avoid losing everything if there is a flood or fire.
2. **Digital Records**
    - Some people scan papers and keep them in password-protected computer folders or cloud accounts. This can be useful for backups.
    - If you do this, ensure someone you trust knows how to access them.
3. **Emergency Contacts**
    - Write down a list of phone numbers for doctors, insurance agents, the bank, and close relatives.
    - Let a family member or a close friend know where this list is in case of urgent need.

Planning Financial Support for Family

1. **Gifts and Donations**
   - You might choose to give small amounts of money to children, grandchildren, or a preferred cause while you are alive.
   - Check any rules about taxes on gifts above certain limits, especially if you plan to give larger sums.
2. **Education Funds**
   - If you want to help grandkids with college, you could set up special accounts (like 529 plans in some places) that might offer tax advantages.
   - This ensures the money is used for education, and you can contribute when you can afford it.
3. **Joint Accounts**
   - Some older adults put an adult child's name on a bank account to handle bills easily if needed.
   - However, note that this can give that child legal ownership of the funds. In addition, other children might feel left out.
   - A POA might be a cleaner solution if your goal is just for them to help with payments.
4. **Leaving Specific Items**
   - If you have special heirlooms, you can list them in your will or a personal letter indicating who should receive them.
   - Communicating your plans beforehand can help loved ones understand your reasoning and reduce conflicts.

Finding Trusted Help

1. **Financial Planners**
   - These experts can review your budget, suggest ways to invest safely, and create a retirement cash-flow plan.
   - Look for someone who explains things in plain language, discloses fees clearly, and has experience working with older clients.
2. **Accountants or Tax Preparers**
   - If taxes feel confusing, especially with retirement incomes or multiple accounts, these professionals can guide you through forms and help you avoid penalties.
   - They might also spot tax credits or deductions you did not know you qualified for.

3. **Eldercare or Legal Aid Groups**
   - Nonprofit groups sometimes offer free advice on basic legal issues like wills or POA forms.
   - They can also point you to local resources for financial support if you face hardship.
4. **Bank or Credit Union Staff**
   - Local bankers might help set up automatic bill pay, open special savings accounts, or explain loan options in a calm setting.
   - They can also share tips on staying secure (for instance, adding alerts for unusual account activity).

Preparing for the Unexpected

1. **Emergency Contacts and Plans**
   - Note who should be called if something sudden happens. This could be a trusted neighbor, a family member in town, or a close friend.
   - Keep this list somewhere obvious, like on the fridge or inside a phone book near the telephone.
2. **Backup Power of Attorney**
   - Sometimes, the main person named in a POA might be unavailable when needed. Naming a backup ensures there is a second option.
   - This can prevent delays in paying bills or making medical decisions.
3. **Automatic Bill Payments**
   - Many utilities or insurance companies let you pay from your bank account automatically. This can prevent missed due dates if you are away or in the hospital.
   - Just remember to keep track, so you do not lose track of account changes.
4. **Plan for Pets**
   - If you have pets, consider who will care for them if you become unable to do so. Write down instructions about feeding, vet care, or medication.
   - Talk to the person you trust, so they agree and know where to find supplies.

Staying Organized

1. **Create a File System**
   - You can have sections for bank statements, insurance details, health documents, and personal papers like a will. Label them clearly.
   - Keep it simple: store all finance-related items in one cabinet or box so you do not lose anything.
2. **Use a Notebook or Planner**
   - Write down bill due dates, any upcoming doctor's appointment fees, or changes in insurance.
   - This can be a paper planner or a digital calendar, whichever you find easiest.
3. **Update Often**
   - Each month or two, review your finances. Are there new bills? Have you canceled a service?
   - Doing small checks along the way is better than waiting a whole year and feeling overwhelmed.
4. **Share Key Details**
   - If you trust a close family member, let them know about your system. In an emergency, they can pick up where you left off.
   - Even a quick talk about "where the bills and documents are" can spare loved ones confusion later.

Encouraging a Mindset of Security

1. **Set Realistic Goals**
   - You do not have to save large amounts at once. Consistent small steps can build a safety net over time.
   - Paying off a small debt or setting aside a bit extra each month can lead to progress.
2. **Celebrate Progress, Gently**
   - If you reduce credit card balances or sign your first will, acknowledge it as a positive achievement.
   - A calm sense of satisfaction can keep you motivated to handle the next financial or legal step.
3. **Learn New Things**

- The world of finance and law can feel complex, but resources (like library books, simple online articles, or local workshops) can teach the basics.
- Asking questions is always okay. Experts are there to help you understand.

4. **Talk Openly**
   - If you feel worried about money or legal topics, try not to keep it bottled up.
   - Share with family, friends, or a professional. Sometimes, just airing concerns helps find solutions faster.

CHAPTER 16: PLANNING FOR RETIREMENT AND WORK OPTIONS

Retirement often means leaving a full-time job, yet it can open up fresh possibilities. Some older adults stop working entirely, while others prefer a mix of part-time jobs, freelance tasks, or side activities that bring in a bit of extra income. For many, the idea of retirement also ties into lifestyle choices, like whether to move closer to family or try living in a smaller home. In this chapter, we will explore ways to plan for retirement and, if desired, remain in the workforce in a manner that fits personal goals. We will avoid repeating health or social tips from earlier chapters, focusing instead on practical ways to organize retirement steps, consider job options, and find meaning in this new stage of life.

The Meaning of Retirement

1. **A Shift in Routine**
    - For years, people might have gone to a job daily, following a set schedule. Retirement can mean freedom from that routine, but it can also leave a gap if you are not sure how to fill your days.
    - Some retirees enjoy having more time to rest, while others worry about feeling bored or missing the sense of purpose from a job.
2. **Adjusting Financial Habits**
    - During work life, a person often receives regular paychecks. In retirement, income may come from Social Security, pensions, or retirement savings, which might feel different.
    - Budgeting might shift to ensure money lasts throughout the rest of life.
3. **Opportunity for Exploration**
    - Retirement can free up hours to explore interests set aside in the past: painting, learning a language, or reading.
    - It can also open space for deeper family involvement, like helping care for grandkids or traveling to see relatives.
4. **Flexible Approaches**
    - Not everyone retires at the same age or in the same way. Some reduce work hours slowly, easing into retirement, while others pick a date and stop completely.
    - Finding what feels right for you is the main goal.

Retirement is not just about finances. It is also about daily structure, personal identity, and how you want to spend your time.

Basics of Retirement Planning

1. **Check Your Income Sources**
   - List possible streams of income: Social Security, pensions from past employers, annuities, retirement accounts like IRAs or 401(k)s, or personal savings.
   - You can estimate how much you will receive each month to see if it covers living costs.
2. **Decide on a Retirement Age**
   - People often choose 62, 65, or 67 because of Social Security or Medicare eligibility. But some work longer or retire earlier.
   - Stopping work too soon might reduce certain benefits. Working longer might give time to save more.
3. **Estimate Expenses**
   - Retirement can change some costs. You might spend less on commuting or work clothes, but more on hobbies or travel.
   - Health-related expenses can rise, so including a buffer in your budget helps avoid surprises.
4. **Consider Housing Choices**
   - Some retirees downsize to smaller places to lower costs and upkeep. Others stay in their current home if it suits them well.
   - Think about whether you want to live near kids or in a community built for seniors with amenities.
5. **Plan for Healthcare**
   - If you retire before official retirement age, ensure you have health insurance coverage.
   - Review how Medicare (or local equivalent programs) works, what it covers, and if you need extra policies for prescriptions or other services.
6. **Test Your Plan**
   - Try living on your expected retirement income for a few months while still working. This can show if your estimates are realistic or if adjustments are needed.
   - It might reveal that you need to save more, or that you can comfortably retire sooner than planned.

Deciding Whether to Keep Working

1. **Reasons to Stay Employed**
    - You may enjoy your job. Some older adults find it energizing and prefer to stay active in the workforce.
    - Additional income can bolster savings or pay for fun extras like short local trips or family gifts.
    - Certain jobs offer health insurance or other benefits that can be valuable.
2. **Cutting Back Hours**
    - Instead of a full stop, some reduce hours or move into a part-time role. This can ease the transition into retirement while still providing a steady paycheck.
    - If the employer agrees, a phased retirement option might balance personal free time and a continued sense of purpose.
3. **Changing Careers**
    - Some older adults feel ready for a new field. Perhaps teaching a skill they have, or shifting to a role with less stress.
    - You can look for job training programs aimed at mature workers. Taking short courses online can open new opportunities.
4. **Gig or Freelance Work**
    - If you have a marketable talent—like writing, consulting, sewing, or carpentry—you might offer services on a freelance basis.
    - This route typically provides flexible hours, though you will need to keep track of business expenses and maybe pay self-employment taxes.
5. **Seasonal Jobs**
    - Helping during holiday rushes or at certain tourist spots in peak season can bring in income without a year-round commitment.
    - This can be appealing if you want variety but do not need constant work.

Practical Steps for Job Hunting in Later Life

1. **Refresh Your Resume**
    - Even if you have decades of experience, keep the format short and highlight your key skills.

- Online job applications often require digital copies. You might need help scanning or formatting your resume for e-submissions.
2. **Look for Age-Friendly Employers**
    - Some companies or community programs value older workers for reliability and experience.
    - Explore job boards aimed at seniors, or ask local senior centers if they have listings.
3. **Practice Interview Skills**
    - If you have not interviewed in a while, consider doing a mock interview with a friend.
    - Prepare answers showing you are flexible, motivated, and eager to learn new methods if needed.
4. **Be Honest About Physical Limits**
    - If a job needs lifting heavy boxes or standing all day, see if your body can handle it. If not, search for positions that suit your comfort level.
    - Let potential employers know if you need minor adjustments, like a stool for sitting or flexible hours for medical appointments.
5. **Online Networking**
    - Some older adults use social media or professional sites (like LinkedIn) to connect with former colleagues and find leads.
    - Keep your profile updated and mention the kind of role you are seeking. You might be surprised who reaches out.

Balancing Work and Personal Life in Retirement

1. **Set Boundaries**
    - If you continue working, decide how many hours you are comfortable giving. Overworking can reduce the benefits of retirement, such as rest or personal projects.
    - Inform your boss or clients about your availability. This keeps expectations in check.
2. **Plan Leisure Time**
    - If you want to travel or enjoy new hobbies, mark them on a calendar. This ensures that work does not take over your retirement.
    - A balanced schedule can keep you energized rather than drained.
3. **Check Income Effects**

- If you take Social Security early and earn above a certain amount, your benefits might be reduced until you reach full retirement age. Understand these rules to avoid surprises.
- Some pensions have limits on earnings from certain jobs, so confirm whether extra income will affect pension payouts.
4. **Prioritize Health**
    - Working in older age can be fulfilling, but be mindful of any physical or mental stress.
    - If a job's demands are too much, it might be time to cut back or pick a gentler option.

Considering Volunteer or Community Roles

1. **Why Volunteer?**
    - Some retirees do not need extra income but still want a sense of purpose and regular activity. Volunteering can fill that gap.
    - You can meet new people, learn new tasks, and feel good about helping your neighborhood.
2. **Choosing an Area**
    - Think about what matters to you. Animals, children's education, libraries, or hospital support are common volunteer fields.
    - Local community centers or websites might list volunteer openings.
3. **Mixing Flexibility with Structure**
    - Some volunteer roles ask for a set day or hours each week, while others let you come when you can.
    - Pick an arrangement that matches your energy and personal schedule.
4. **Personal Growth**
    - Volunteering can sharpen your skills, whether it is organizing items, talking with people, or planning small events.
    - You might discover hidden strengths or new interests. This keeps the mind active and promotes a sense of connection.

Exploring Small Business Possibilities

1. **Turn Hobbies into Income**

- If you like baking, crafts, or home repairs, you might offer products or services to neighbors.
- Setting fair prices and letting people know you are available can gradually bring in customers.

2. **Online Marketplaces**
    - Some older adults sell handmade goods or collectibles on internet platforms. This can reach many buyers beyond your local area.
    - Be cautious about shipping costs and learn how to photograph items clearly if you are selling crafts or art.
3. **Local Partnerships**
    - If handling a business alone feels daunting, team up with a friend who shares your interests.
    - You might rent a small booth at a craft fair or a farmer's market together, splitting costs and tasks.
4. **Staying Realistic**
    - A small business can be fun, but it involves duties like record-keeping, paying taxes, and customer service.
    - Decide if you want a casual hobby that covers some costs or if you aim for a larger profit. This helps manage time and stress levels.

Lifestyle Choices in Retirement

1. **Downsizing or Relocating**
    - Moving to a smaller home can free up money from the sale of a larger house, potentially covering some retirement expenses.
    - Some retirees move closer to family or pick a setting with warm weather and recreational activities.
2. **Senior Living Communities**
    - These communities can range from independent apartments to places that offer help with daily tasks.
    - If you like being around people of a similar age or want amenities (like group events, meal plans), this might be an option.
3. **Staying Put (Aging in Place)**
    - Others want to remain in their longtime home. In that case, consider if you need to adjust the home for safety—like installing grab bars or a ramp.
    - Hiring occasional help for chores or yard work might be worth exploring.

4. **Travel and Exploration**
    - With fewer job commitments, you can take short trips to nearby places of interest.
    - Some older adults enjoy group travel tours geared toward seniors, offering guided experiences and easy transportation.

Social Connections for Retirees

1. **Joining Clubs or Groups**
    - Retirement often means more time for group activities, such as walking clubs, book clubs, or community singing groups.
    - This can offset any loneliness if you no longer see coworkers daily.
2. **Skill-Sharing**
    - If you have expertise—like cooking or carpentry—offering short lessons to neighbors or hosting small workshops can nurture social bonds.
    - Community centers might provide space for classes if you want to teach.
3. **Online Meetups**
    - If mobility is tricky, virtual clubs or chat groups can connect you with people who share similar interests.
    - Some retirees find new friends across the country or even the world.
4. **Multigenerational Interaction**
    - Volunteering at schools, libraries, or youth clubs can introduce you to younger generations, helping both sides learn from each other.
    - This variety in social contacts can keep life interesting and reduce isolation.

Financial Checks During Retirement

1. **Regular Budget Reviews**
    - Expenses and income can change. Maybe you took on a part-time role or faced new medical bills.
    - Checking your finances every few months keeps you on track, so you do not run short later.

2. **Managing Required Minimum Distributions (RMDs)**
   - If you have certain retirement accounts, you may be required to withdraw a minimum sum each year once you reach a certain age (depending on local laws).
   - Failure to do so could result in penalties, so stay aware of the required amounts and deadlines.
3. **Insurance Reevaluations**
   - If you have life insurance, compare the premiums to your current needs. Possibly, you no longer require as much coverage.
   - If your health has changed, explore whether you need different supplements for medical insurance.
4. **Small Adjustments**
   - If funds look tight, you can reduce some non-essential spending or consider a short-term seasonal job.
   - If you have extra, you might save more or treat yourself to a special outing or an improvement in your living space.

Time Management and Purpose

1. **Create a Loose Daily Structure**
   - Waking up with no plan might feel overwhelming. Having a casual schedule—like breakfast, a walk, a hobby session—can offer a sense of direction.
   - Leave room for flexibility if a friend calls or if you decide to run an errand.
2. **Pursue Passions**
   - Think back to old interests you paused while working, like painting, fishing, or learning an instrument. Devote consistent time to them now.
   - These personal projects can enrich retirement and keep the mind engaged.
3. **Set Small Goals**
   - Maybe aim to read a certain number of books each month or learn basic phrases in a new language.
   - Reaching these goals provides a sense of fulfillment and keeps life meaningful.
4. **Combine Service and Leisure**

- Some retirees volunteer a few days a week, then reserve other days for relaxation or family.
- This blend can prevent boredom while keeping stress in check.

Handling Emotional Changes

1. **Identity Shifts**
    - Many people define themselves by their jobs. Retirement can bring questions like, "Who am I without my work?"
    - Exploring hobbies, social roles, or spiritual practices can help rebuild a sense of identity.
2. **Loneliness or Boredom**
    - If coworkers were your main social circle, it can feel lonely once you leave. Seek new contacts in clubs, churches, or local gatherings.
    - If physical restrictions limit going out, invite friends over or consider online meetups.
3. **Rest vs. Activity**
    - Some older adults feel they must fill every moment to remain useful, while others slow down more than they want.
    - Balance rest and activity in a way that feels right. There is no single path all retirees must follow.
4. **Talking with Others**
    - Sharing ups and downs with peers who are also retired can ease your mind.
    - If deep sadness persists, a mental health counselor or a trusted community leader might offer guidance.

Future Directions

1. **Planning for Later Stages**
    - As time passes, you may need more help with daily tasks. Think about whether you prefer home-based care, moving in with family, or a senior residence if that time comes.
    - Discuss these ideas openly with family so that everyone is prepared.
2. **Celebrating Milestones Gently**

- Even though we are avoiding certain words (like ones we are not supposed to use here), it is okay to take note of personal achievements. For instance, finishing your first year of retirement might feel satisfying.
- You might share a nice meal with loved ones or send a note to a friend, marking the progress.

3. **Giving Yourself Room to Adapt**
    - Retirement does not have to be an instant, unchanging phase. You may start with one plan, adjust if money or health changes, and adapt again if new opportunities appear.
    - Stay open to learning new skills, especially if technology or local services shift.
4. **Inspiring Others**
    - Sometimes, older adults can encourage younger folks by showing that later life can be active, interesting, and full of creativity.
    - Sharing stories about your own path could guide friends or family members who worry about their own retirement down the line.

CHAPTER 17: EMOTIONAL HEALTH AND STAYING POSITIVE

Growing older brings many changes—some pleasant and some more challenging. While physical health is important, so is emotional well-being. Feeling positive or at ease can help in daily life and in coping with shifts that come with age. Emotions can influence how a person thinks, makes decisions, and relates to others. In this chapter, we will discuss ways to keep a more balanced mood, handle negative feelings, and find methods to support an overall sense of well-being. We will avoid repeating earlier tips on stress and socializing in depth, focusing on fresh ideas for emotional resilience and maintaining a brighter outlook.

Understanding Emotional Well-Being in Older Age

1. **Normal Emotional Shifts**
    - As life changes—such as retirement, new living arrangements, or losing people close to us—feelings can be affected.
    - Some older adults might notice they experience quiet moments of reflection more often. Others may find new joys in simple routines.
2. **Positive vs. Negative Emotions**
    - Feeling calm or content often indicates emotional balance, while feeling down might signal the need for extra support or a slight change in routine.
    - Occasional sadness or anxiety can be normal, but if these feelings last a long time or interrupt daily tasks, it might be a sign to seek help.
3. **Influence of Physical Health**
    - Physical discomfort (like chronic pain or low energy) can reduce a person's mood. Likewise, emotional distress might lower energy or affect sleep.
    - Addressing physical concerns can, in turn, boost emotional health and vice versa.
4. **Ongoing Adaptation**
    - Emotional well-being is not a one-time achievement—it shifts day by day. Some days feel great, others are harder. Learning ways to handle these swings can make everyday life more comfortable.

Emotions are part of who we are at any age. Older adults can benefit from learning fresh methods to handle feelings in supportive, healthy ways.

Finding Meaning and Purpose

1. **Reflecting on Life Experiences**
   - Older adults have a lifetime of stories—challenges faced, lessons learned, skills developed. Looking back at these can remind a person of their resilience.
   - Sharing memories with trusted individuals or writing them down can strengthen self-esteem and bring clarity to what feels important today.
2. **Setting New Goals**
   - Goals do not need to be huge. They can be simple tasks, such as finishing a small craft project or reading a certain number of books in a month.
   - Having aims—whether small or large—can create a sense of forward movement and positivity.
3. **Passing on Knowledge**
   - Teaching a younger neighbor how to fix a minor home problem or guiding a friend in a hobby can give a sense of helping others.
   - This exchange can remind an older adult that their experience and insights matter.
4. **Embracing Small Acts of Kindness**
   - Simple gestures, like offering a friendly word to a neighbor, can create a personal feeling of warmth.
   - Even small steps—like writing a supportive note to someone having a tough time—can lead to positive feelings about oneself and the world.

Purpose can take many forms. It might involve volunteering, creative pursuits, or quietly enjoying a pastime that makes each day feel meaningful.

Tools for a More Balanced Mood

1. **Breathing Exercises**
   - Though we have mentioned stress relief in other sections, we have not focused on a fresh angle. Here, an older adult can practice

slow, steady breathing to help soothe sudden emotional upsets, such as frustration or brief sadness.
    - A simple approach: Inhale slowly for four counts, hold for a moment, and exhale gently for four counts. Repeat a few times to feel calmer.
2. **Grounding Through the Senses**
    - If negative thoughts swirl, turning attention to the senses—such as noticing the color of a nearby flower or feeling the texture of a blanket—can bring the mind back to the present moment.
    - This technique offers a short mental break from worries or regrets.
3. **Journaling Emotions**
    - Writing down feelings—even if it is just a few sentences—helps release them from the mind.
    - A small notebook by the bedside can be used in the morning or evening to jot down thoughts, which can provide insight into mood patterns over time.
4. **Visual Reminders**
    - Placing uplifting words or a photo of a peaceful place on the fridge can spark a gentle positive feeling whenever it is seen.
    - Some older adults use small sticky notes with simple affirmations like, "I can handle today," where they will see them often.

Emotional calm is not about ignoring or denying hard feelings. It is about having methods to pause, center oneself, and decide what steps to take.

Handling Loss and Grief

1. **Recognizing Grief**
    - Loss can mean losing a partner, a friend, or even a pet. It can also come from losing a sense of ability or independence.
    - Grief is personal: some feel numb, others cry or feel restless. There is no single correct way to grieve.
2. **Giving Yourself Time**
    - Grief does not vanish overnight. It can lessen gradually or resurface on significant dates.
    - Being patient with emotional ups and downs is crucial. Rushing oneself to feel "normal" can add pressure.

3. **Memorial Activities**
    - Doing something in memory of a loved one—like planting a small tree or setting out a framed photo—can gently honor their place in one's life.
    - Sharing stories about positive memories can bring both sadness and comfort at the same time.
4. **Support Systems**
    - Talking to a counselor or a grief support group can help process these emotions.
    - If in-person groups are not available, phone or online support can still offer human connection and understanding.

Loss is a natural part of living a full life. Acknowledging it rather than pushing it away can help older adults eventually find a renewed sense of emotional balance.

Steadying Negative Thought Patterns

1. **Awareness of Inner Talk**
    - Sometimes, an older adult might silently repeat discouraging messages, like "I am too old for that" or "No one cares what I think."
    - Noticing these thoughts is the first step—recognizing that they might not be facts but rather unhelpful habits of the mind.
2. **Replacing with Balanced Alternatives**
    - It is not about ignoring problems but about shifting "I cannot" to something gentler like, "I can try, even if it is not perfect."
    - This approach opens the door for possibility rather than final defeat.
3. **Focusing on Achievements**
    - It can help to list small successes of the day: finishing a chore, writing a letter, or learning a bit of new information.
    - These little wins remind an older adult that they are still capable of moving forward and handling new tasks.
4. **Recognizing Exaggerations**
    - Terms like "always" and "never" can creep in, making problems seem larger. Thinking "I always mess up" or "I never get calls from anyone" can be more extreme than reality.
    - Checking for facts—maybe you do get a call every now and then—can soften such blanket statements.

Rewiring negative thinking does not mean ignoring genuine problems. It is about seeing them in a more balanced way that can encourage solutions and hope.

Encouraging a Cheerful Mindset

1. **Daily Gratitude Moments**
    - Writing a short list of things to be thankful for each day can help highlight the positive side of life: a sunny morning, a quick call from a friend, or a tasty meal.
    - Even on tough days, searching for one small good detail can brighten mood.
2. **Creative Expression**
    - Activities like coloring simple pages or arranging flowers can nurture a gentle sense of delight.
    - Creativity does not demand fancy skills. It is about exploring shapes, colors, or sounds in a playful manner.
3. **Laughter and Lightness**
    - Watching a funny, uplifting show or rereading a humorous book can offer a break from serious concerns.
    - Sharing laughs with another person fosters connection. If alone, even remembering a funny moment can bring a smile.
4. **Healthful Humor**
    - Joking at one's own expense can be okay if it is mild, but be mindful if it becomes self-putdowns. The aim is to maintain a kindly humor, not to degrade oneself.

Positivity can serve as a cushion against life's bumps. Finding small joys or silly moments can help an older adult stay more mentally flexible and less weighed down by worries.

Accepting Help and Guidance

1. **Recognizing When to Seek Support**
    - If sadness, worry, or anger seems constant, or if daily tasks feel too overwhelming, talking to a professional or a supportive confidant might help.
    - There is no shame in reaching out. It shows self-awareness and willingness to improve.

2. **Possible Avenues**
   - **Counseling**: A mental health counselor can offer practical tools to handle ongoing emotional difficulties.
   - **Groups**: Some communities have small gatherings where older adults talk about life, share stories, and learn from each other.
   - **Hotlines**: If someone feels extremely low in the middle of the night, calling a trusted help line might bring calm.
3. **Light Medication**
   - For some, a doctor might suggest mild medication to help with persistent low mood or anxiety.
   - It is wise to discuss any worries about side effects or interactions with other medicines. A careful approach can ensure safety.
4. **Spiritual or Community Leaders**
   - If religion or spiritual practice is part of a person's life, a trusted leader can offer encouragement, read uplifting texts, or share comforting words.
   - This guidance can help an older adult feel less alone in facing emotional hurdles.

Seeking help is a sign of inner strength. Knowing personal limits and finding resources can ease burdens and restore a sense of balance.

Nurturing Self-Esteem

1. **Acceptance of Changes**
   - Bodies and abilities can shift with age, but that does not lessen personal worth. Self-esteem can stay strong by focusing on what one can do rather than what is lost.
   - Adjusting activities—like cooking seated if standing is tough—can empower older adults to continue doing what they love.
2. **Self-Compassion**
   - Treating oneself with kindness is important. If a project takes longer than before, that is fine. If there is a need for more rest, that too is acceptable.
   - Negative self-criticism drains energy. A gentle approach reminds us we are still learning at every stage of life.
3. **Taking Pride in Small Actions**
   - Completing a puzzle, organizing a drawer, or figuring out a new device can feel gratifying, no matter how small the task.

- A sense of accomplishment does not require big achievements—tiny daily wins matter too.
4. **Positive Body Image**
    - Lines on the face or gray hair can be viewed as signs of experience rather than flaws. Focusing on what the body can do (e.g., walk a bit each day, see loved ones) can keep perspective.
    - Wearing clothes that feel comfortable and pleasing can boost mood and self-confidence.

Self-esteem grows when someone sees themselves as capable, regardless of what changes life brings.

Strengthening Emotional Resilience

1. **Learning New Skills**
    - Trying fresh activities—like a new hobby or a tech tool—can show older adults they can still adapt.
    - Being open to small challenges, from following a new recipe to using a phone app, can build mental flexibility.
2. **Practicing Forgiveness**
    - Holding onto past resentments can hurt emotional well-being. While not always simple, letting go of grudges or regrets can free a person's mind.
    - This does not mean forgetting, but deciding not to let old hurts control present feelings.
3. **Balancing Alone Time and Connection**
    - Quiet moments can be soothing, allowing reflection or rest. But isolation can grow if alone time becomes too frequent.
    - Ensuring some form of contact—through calls, letters, or visits—can keep emotional resilience steadier.
4. **Adapting to Routine Disruptions**
    - Unexpected changes, like a sudden home repair or a shift in a friend's availability, can be jarring.
    - Resilient older adults practice calm problem-solving, reminding themselves they have handled similar issues before.

Resilience does not mean ignoring challenges; it means bouncing back and staying rooted in hope despite them.

Emotional Challenges Tied to Physical Changes

1. **Vision or Hearing Loss**
    - Losing some vision or hearing can lead to frustration, embarrassment, or feeling left out of conversations.
    - Seeking tools—like bigger text, hearing aids, or quieter meeting spots—can help restore confidence and reduce emotional strain.
2. **Decreased Mobility**
    - If walking or climbing stairs is harder, older adults might need to limit certain outings, which can spark sadness or worry.
    - Finding new ways to engage—like shorter walks, using canes or walkers, or planning rides—can reduce emotional burdens from mobility limits.
3. **Sleep Disruptions**
    - Changes in sleep patterns might lead to irritability or low mood during the day.
    - Approaches like a gentle bedtime routine or speaking with a healthcare provider about underlying causes can ease this strain.
4. **Chronic Pain**
    - Lingering pain can make any emotion feel heavier. It is normal to feel discouraged when physical discomfort persists.
    - Exploring pain management strategies—like mild relaxation methods, safe medication, or comfortable positioning—can help keep emotional health steadier.

Physical changes do not have to rule emotional well-being. Adjusting routines and using available aids can help older adults remain emotionally balanced even with bodily shifts.

Handling Emotional Overload

1. **Signs of Overload**
    - Losing temper easily, feeling constantly on edge, forgetting simple tasks, or feeling mentally numb can suggest emotional strain is too high.
    - Physical signs might include headaches, tense muscles, or a queasy stomach with no other explanation.
2. **Immediate Calming Methods**
    - Step away from the situation—if safe—and try a quick slow-breathing exercise.

- If possible, splash cool water on your face or take a brief seat outdoors to reset the mind.
3. **Sharing Feelings Quickly**
    - Talking with a friend or family member, even for five minutes, can help discharge some tension.
    - If no one is available, writing a quick note or message to yourself about the cause of overload can lessen its intensity.
4. **Long-Term Solutions**
    - Consider adjusting routines or tasks that cause repeated overload. Breaking chores into smaller steps might help.
    - If a certain trigger cannot be avoided (like medical appointments), plan rest or calming breaks afterward to regroup.

Overload is a sign that daily strategies might need tweaking. By making small changes or seeking a bit of help, older adults can regain a healthier emotional state.

Celebrating Cheerful Moments with Others

(We will avoid using the exact word we are not supposed to use—replacing it with "marking" or "appreciating," for instance.)

1. **Marking Good Occasions**
    - A family birthday or a friend's small victory can be recognized with a simple gesture: a card, a phone call, or a homemade treat.
    - This shared recognition spreads positivity and fosters closeness.
2. **Appreciating Personal Wins**
    - Whether it is finishing a puzzle or managing a tough conversation calmly, acknowledging these positives can make them feel more special.
    - Some older adults might keep a small note of personal achievements each week to reinforce confidence.
3. **Teamwork in Small Gatherings**
    - If friends come by, propose a small group game or collaborative cooking session. Working together can spark smiles and supportive conversations.
    - It keeps the focus on fellowship rather than daily problems.
4. **Gentle Observances**

- Even lighting a small candle for a moment to honor a good memory can give a sense of quiet positivity.
- These little acts do not have to be big parties; they just remind us that positive feelings deserve recognition too.

Honoring good moments underscores the fact that, alongside life's challenges, joys still bloom at any age.

When Professional Emotional Care Is Needed

1. **Signs That Help Is Urgent**
    - Thoughts of self-harm, giving away possessions suddenly, or a deep sense of hopelessness might be urgent signals.
    - Marked changes in behavior—like not eating, refusing to get out of bed, or severe confusion—also suggest immediate professional evaluation.
2. **What to Expect from Therapy**
    - A counselor or psychiatrist will often ask questions about mood, daily routines, and concerns. They work with older adults to develop manageable steps toward improvement.
    - Sometimes they may suggest talk therapy, group sessions, or short-term medication support.
3. **Involving Family or Caregivers**
    - If an older adult struggles to remember to attend appointments or take medication, supportive relatives can help with scheduling and gentle reminders.
    - This team approach often leads to better outcomes.
4. **Hospital or Crisis Care**
    - In rare cases, if emotional distress is severe, a brief hospital stay or crisis intervention might be necessary to ensure safety.
    - Medical staff can adjust medication, offer counseling, and stabilize mental health before the individual returns home.

Recognizing that emotional pain can be as critical as physical illness is key. There is no shame in using professional resources when needed.

CHAPTER 18: GUARDING AGAINST COMMON ILLNESSES

With age, the body's ability to fight off infections and other health issues can change. While many older adults stay reasonably healthy, certain illnesses become more likely or harder to bounce back from. Knowing how to reduce risks and handle minor sicknesses before they become serious can be a big help. In this chapter, we will look at ways to guard against frequent illnesses, maintain a cleaner environment, and remain mindful of small warning signs. We will not repeat topics about daily movement or nutrition in detail, focusing instead on strategies specifically aimed at preventing or managing common health challenges in older adulthood.

Why Older Adults May Be More Vulnerable

1. **Immune System Shifts**
   - Over the years, the immune system might not respond as quickly, making older adults more open to infections from viruses or bacteria.
   - Healing can also take longer if cuts or illnesses arise.
2. **Chronic Conditions**
   - Some individuals deal with ongoing health issues like diabetes or heart problems, which can weaken the body's defenses.
   - Certain medicines for these conditions may reduce immunity or mask early signs of infection.
3. **Limited Mobility**
   - If mobility is reduced, it can be harder to get regular fresh air or do chores like cleaning thoroughly, which can lead to environments where germs spread.
   - Less physical movement can also mean the body's circulation is slower, potentially affecting how swiftly it combats illness.
4. **Close Living Arrangements**
   - Retirement communities or shared homes can be cozy, but germs may spread faster in group settings.
   - Careful hygiene is even more important in these environments.

Still, there are many ways to lower these risks. A blend of simple caution, smart habits, and timely check-ups can help older adults ward off many of the common health threats.

Basic Hygiene Practices

1. **Regular Hand Washing**
   - Washing hands with mild soap and warm water for about 20 seconds can remove germs picked up from door handles, groceries, or other surfaces.
   - Dry hands thoroughly because dampness can allow bacteria to linger.
2. **Hand Sanitizer**
   - If soap and water are not handy, an alcohol-based sanitizer can kill most germs.
   - Keep a small bottle in a purse or near the front door to use after returning from errands.
3. **Avoid Touching Face Excessively**
   - Many illnesses enter through the nose, mouth, or eyes. Keeping hands away from the face lowers this risk.
   - If you must touch your face (like adjusting glasses), try to wash or sanitize hands first.
4. **Tissue and Mask Use**
   - If sneezing or coughing, a tissue or the inside of the elbow helps stop droplets from spreading.
   - In crowded spaces, wearing a simple face mask may protect against airborne germs, especially during cold or flu season.

These simple steps might seem obvious, but they remain some of the best defenses against everyday illnesses.

Keeping the Home Environment Safer

1. **Routine Cleaning**
   - Disinfect surfaces that are touched often—like doorknobs, light switches, and remote controls.

- A basic household cleaner or diluted bleach solution can kill many germs.
2. **Kitchen Hygiene**
    - Wash fruits and vegetables before eating, and keep raw meat away from other foods.
    - Wipe countertops and cutting boards with soapy water, and dry them well to reduce bacterial growth.
3. **Bathroom Care**
    - Bathrooms can be damp, which helps germs thrive. Hanging towels to dry and using a fan or opening windows can reduce moisture.
    - Cleaning sinks, toilet seats, and tubs regularly helps stop harmful microbes from settling in.
4. **Ventilation**
    - Fresh air can carry away stale air that might hold viruses or molds. Opening a window for a short time each day, if weather allows, can boost air quality.
    - If air pollution is high in your region, consider using an air filter indoors.

A clean home does not have to be sterile, but reducing clutter and moisture can keep germs from finding easy hiding spots.

Seasonal Illness Tips

1. **Colds and Flu**
    - Older adults can be hit harder by common colds or flu, which may lead to complications like pneumonia.
    - Annual flu shots are usually recommended to reduce the risk of severe symptoms.
2. **Pneumonia**
    - Vaccinations exist to help prevent certain types of pneumonia, a lung infection that can be serious in older adults.
    - If a cold or flu lasts longer than usual or breathing feels heavy, it is wise to see a healthcare professional to rule out pneumonia.
3. **Allergies vs. Infections**
    - Sometimes a runny nose or cough could be from allergies rather than a virus. Learning to spot the difference can save worry.

- If symptoms persist or worsen quickly, a check-up may be needed.
4. **Extreme Weather**
    - In very hot or cold months, the body might be less able to regulate temperature, leading to stress on the immune system.
    - Staying hydrated in heat and wearing layered clothing in cold can help the body remain stable and better able to resist illnesses.

Seasonal challenges change, but being ready with the right protective measures can keep minor bugs from turning into bigger problems.

Recognizing Early Signs of Illness

1. **Fever or Chills**
    - A mild increase in temperature might not always be noticed by older adults, especially if they cannot sense changes well or take medications that mask fever.
    - If you feel unusually cold or warm, checking your temperature with a thermometer can clarify if you have a fever.
2. **Unusual Tiredness**
    - A sudden wave of fatigue could indicate the start of an infection, especially if it is paired with body aches or slight headaches.
    - Rest can help the immune system do its job, but if fatigue is severe or unrelenting, contacting a healthcare professional can be wise.
3. **Cough or Sore Throat**
    - While a small cough might just be a dry throat, a persistent or worsening one may mean a respiratory infection.
    - Paying attention to how it changes over a day or two can guide when to seek assistance.
4. **Upset Stomach**
    - Nausea, vomiting, or diarrhea can occur for many reasons, but in older adults, dehydration can happen more quickly.
    - Drinking clear fluids or an electrolyte solution can prevent serious fluid loss, and a doctor might need to be consulted if symptoms last.

Spotting these clues early allows an older adult to rest, use home care remedies if appropriate, and avoid letting something small become severe.

Doctor and Dental Visits

1. **Regular Check-Ups**
   - Seeing a doctor for routine health assessments can find issues before they grow. This might include checking blood pressure, sugar levels, or other markers.
   - Vaccinations against flu, pneumonia, shingles, or other preventable illnesses might be updated during these visits.
2. **Dental Health**
   - Mouth infections can spread bacteria to other parts of the body. Keeping teeth and gums clean is vital.
   - Regular dental exams can catch problems early, such as tooth decay or gum disease, which might otherwise lead to pain or infection.
3. **Honesty About Symptoms**
   - Telling healthcare providers about even small changes (like unusual tiredness or mild dizziness) can help them see patterns.
   - Bringing a list of questions to appointments ensures you address concerns without forgetting.
4. **Medication Check-Ins**
   - Some medicines can dull immunity or interact badly with new drugs. Reviewing prescriptions with a doctor or pharmacist reduces risks.
   - If a certain medicine seems to cause tiredness or other side effects, mentioning it can prompt a switch to a safer option.

Staying current with doctor and dental visits is not just about addressing existing issues—it is also about preventing new ones and ensuring the body remains as strong as possible.

Preventing Falls and Injuries

Though not exactly an "illness," falls are a major concern among older adults and can lead to hospital stays or infections if injuries occur.

1. **Safe Home Setup**
   - Secure loose rugs, improve lighting in hallways, and consider grab bars in the bathroom. This can stop minor slips from happening.

        ○ Keeping walkways clear of clutter (like shoes or boxes) is also important.
   2. **Shoes and Foot Care**
        ○ Wearing sturdy, well-fitting shoes can provide stability. Avoid floppy slippers or shoes with worn soles.
        ○ Regular foot check-ups can catch toenail issues or infections that might affect balance and comfort.
   3. **Supportive Aids**
        ○ A cane or walker can help with balance if standing feels unsteady. Using them properly (with guidance from a therapist or doctor) can lower the chance of a tumble.
        ○ Some older adults resist mobility aids at first, but they can be a key step in staying safe and independent.
   4. **Immediate Medical Attention After Falls**
        ○ Even if a fall seems minor, a doctor's check might be needed. Hidden injuries or slow-developing complications can arise, especially in older bodies.
        ○ Quick treatment can prevent infections if scrapes or cuts occur during a fall.

Preventing falls is a way of preventing secondary illnesses or complications that might follow an injury.

Care for Skin and Wound Prevention

   1. **Daily Skin Checks**
        ○ Dry or thinning skin can lead to small tears or cracks that become infected if not treated. A quick look at arms, legs, and feet can catch minor cuts early.
        ○ If reaching certain areas is difficult, using a handheld mirror or asking for help might be necessary.
   2. **Gentle Cleansing and Moisturizing**
        ○ Using mild soaps and warm water can protect older skin from dryness. A fragrance-free moisturizer right after bathing helps lock in moisture.
        ○ For those in bed or seated for long periods, occasionally shifting position prevents pressure sores that can become infected.
   3. **Handling Small Cuts**

- Washing a cut gently with soap and clean water, then applying a fresh bandage can keep germs out.
- If redness, swelling, or pain around a wound grows, seeking medical advice promptly is wise.

4. **Nail Trimming**
   - Overly long nails can scratch the skin or cause ingrown nails. Keeping nails trimmed and clean reduces these risks.
   - If vision or hand steadiness is an issue, a podiatrist or a helpful family member can assist.

Preventing wounds and caring for skin is a quiet but crucial way to reduce infection risk, especially for those with reduced mobility.

Food Safety for Illness Prevention

1. **Proper Food Storage**
   - Storing perishable goods in the fridge soon after shopping can prevent bacterial growth.
   - Freezing items that will not be eaten soon can also preserve freshness and safety.
2. **Watching Expiration Dates**
   - Older adults sometimes stock up on foods, but outdated items can harbor dangerous bacteria or mold.
   - Checking labels each week and discarding expired foods helps avoid accidental consumption.
3. **Cooking Meats Thoroughly**
   - Undercooked poultry or meats can carry germs like salmonella. Using a food thermometer ensures the center reaches a safe temperature.
   - Washing hands and surfaces after handling raw meats is essential.
4. **Leftover Guidelines**
   - Leftovers kept too long in the fridge can spoil. As a rule, most cooked items are best eaten within a few days.
   - Reheating foods to steaming hot can kill some bacteria, but do not rely on reheating if the food has been left out for hours.

Safe eating habits are not complicated, but they play a big role in avoiding stomach upsets or more serious infections.

Supplements and Vitamins

1. **Consulting a Professional**
   - While certain vitamins (like Vitamin D or B12) might help some older adults, it is wise to speak with a doctor before starting any supplement.
   - Some supplements can interact with prescriptions or be unnecessary if you get enough nutrients from your meals.
2. **Calcium and Bone Health**
   - Some older adults consider calcium pills to support bone strength. Again, checking with a professional ensures you choose a correct dose.
   - Too much calcium can affect kidneys or other body systems.
3. **Immune-Boosting Claims**
   - Many products claim to boost the immune system, but not all are backed by science. Some might be fine, while others could do harm.
   - A balanced approach of healthy eating and hygiene remains the top method to guard against infections.
4. **Avoid Over-Reliance**
   - Supplements are not a magic shield. They can support the body if used wisely, but they cannot replace careful hygiene, vaccines, or a clean environment.

Mental and Emotional Factors Affecting Illness

1. **Stress Levels**
   - Though we are not discussing stress in depth here, acknowledging that high stress can weaken the body's defenses is relevant.
   - Simple calming practices can keep the immune system more robust.
2. **Loneliness and Health**
   - Feeling isolated sometimes leads to ignoring early signs of illness or skipping care. Having someone check in can prompt timely help.
   - Friendly chats or brief visits encourage older adults to mention small symptoms that might require action.
3. **Motivation for Prevention**

- If a person feels hopeless, they might not bother with hygiene or healthy routines.
- Encouragement from friends or family can renew interest in daily tasks that protect health.

Even emotional well-being ties into how well a person avoids or deals with illnesses, making mental self-care an indirect ally for physical health.

Handling Mild Illness at Home

1. **Rest and Hydration**
    - At the first sign of a minor cold, gentle rest and enough fluids can help the body recover faster.
    - Water, broth, or warm herbal drinks can soothe a throat or help loosen congestion.
2. **Home Remedies**
    - For stuffy noses, inhaling warm steam (perhaps from a bowl of hot water or a warm shower) can offer relief.
    - For mild coughs, sipping honey mixed in warm water or tea might calm the throat. (Check for possible sugar concerns if you have diabetes.)
3. **Safe Use of Over-the-Counter Aids**
    - Some cold or flu medications contain ingredients that may conflict with prescriptions, especially for blood pressure or heart conditions.
    - Reading labels or asking a pharmacist ensures you pick a product that is gentle enough and free of risky interactions.
4. **When to Seek a Doctor**
    - If a mild illness gets worse over two or three days or includes high fever or severe symptoms, it is time for medical help.
    - Trusting one's instincts can be crucial. If you feel something is not right, calling a medical professional is safer than waiting too long.

These home care steps can address small issues, but staying vigilant to warning signs is essential.

Vaccination Options

1. **Annual Flu Shot**
   - This is often recommended for older adults to reduce the impact of seasonal flu. If caught, the illness may be less severe if vaccinated.
   - Usually given in the fall, but can be received any time during flu season.
2. **Pneumococcal Vaccines**
   - These target bacteria that lead to certain types of pneumonia, blood infections, or meningitis. Some older adults might need one or two doses, depending on their history and doctor's guidance.
3. **Shingles Vaccine**
   - Shingles (caused by the same virus as chickenpox) can be painful and more common in older adults. A vaccine can cut down the chance or seriousness of an outbreak.
   - Even if you have had shingles before, a vaccine might help prevent future flare-ups.
4. **Tetanus, Diphtheria, and Pertussis (Tdap)**
   - Boosters for tetanus and diphtheria are often given every 10 years. Adding pertussis coverage helps protect against whooping cough, which can be severe in older adults.

Ensuring vaccines are up to date can shield an older adult from various threats, so discussing these with a healthcare provider is wise.

Recognizing Urgent Signs

1. **Chest Pain**
   - Not all chest pain means a heart attack, but any unusual pressure or tightness should be treated seriously, especially if linked with shortness of breath or dizziness.
2. **Difficulty Breathing**
   - If it suddenly becomes hard to breathe, or breathing is much faster or shallower than normal, it might be an emergency situation.
3. **Confusion or Disorientation**

- Sudden confusion—such as not knowing where you are or who people are—can point to an infection (like a urinary tract infection that spread) or other serious problems.
4. **Severe Headache**
     - An unusual, intense headache, particularly if accompanied by vision changes or trouble speaking, might need immediate care.

Time is critical in these cases. Acting quickly can reduce complications and support better recovery outcomes.

Building a Support Network

1. **Family and Neighbors**
     - Having a contact list with phone numbers for relatives or trustworthy neighbors allows for quick help if you feel unwell.
     - Agreeing to check in at set times can reassure everyone involved.
2. **Local Community Resources**
     - Some communities offer meal deliveries, volunteer ride services to doctor appointments, or friendly call programs.
     - Knowing about these in advance can ease worries when illness pops up.
3. **Online and Phone Helplines**
     - Certain health organizations have lines to answer questions about symptoms or let you speak with a nurse.
     - This is helpful if you are unsure whether to visit a clinic or just rest at home.
4. **Peer Support Groups**
     - Meeting or chatting with people in similar health situations can supply tips on how they manage symptoms or keep their home germ-free.
     - It also helps combat loneliness, which can indirectly guard against illness by keeping morale and motivation higher.

A strong network ensures that if you do get sick, help is not far off, making recovery more likely and safer.

CHAPTER 19: CHECK-UPS AND REGULAR SCREENINGS

As people grow older, regular medical check-ups and screenings become a powerful way to stay ahead of possible health concerns. A check-up is more than just a visit to the doctor when you feel unwell. It can also be a planned meeting to see how your body is doing, spot small problems early, and learn new ways to protect your well-being. Screenings—like certain scans or lab tests—are often part of this routine. They help find signs of illness before symptoms even appear. By taking part in these check-ups and screenings, older adults can improve their odds of enjoying a more comfortable life.

In this chapter, we will look at different check-ups that might matter to older adults, from basic wellness visits to screening programs for hidden problems in the heart, bones, or different organs. We will also share how to prepare for appointments, what to discuss with doctors, and ways to make sure you are getting the care that meets your personal needs. We will avoid repeating previous advice about diet, daily movement, or stress in detail, focusing instead on the check-up process itself, the meaning of key screenings, and tips for using medical appointments as a tool to stay healthier.

Why Check-Ups Matter in Later Life

1. **Catching Problems Early**
    - Some health issues develop quietly and do not cause pain at first. Screenings can detect things like high blood pressure or growths before you notice any changes. Finding them sooner often means treatment can be simpler and more successful.
    - Early detection can help prevent small concerns from turning into big ones. For instance, if a doctor finds high blood sugar early, you might be able to handle it with modest changes and limit the risk of complications later.
2. **Tracking Changes Over Time**
    - The body changes as years go by. What was normal last year might shift slightly this year. Regular check-ups let you and your doctor compare test results and track trends.

- If test numbers move in an unexpected direction, your healthcare provider can react faster, perhaps adjusting medications or suggesting further tests.
3. **Staying Informed**
    - Medical knowledge evolves. New screening tests or updated guidelines can appear. Regular visits help you hear about fresh options that might fit your situation.
    - Doctors can also warn you about any new vaccines you might need or mention medical alerts that could be relevant for older adults.
4. **Providing a Sense of Control**
    - Some people feel uneasy about going to the doctor. But check-ups can also bring calmness once you know your numbers (such as blood pressure, cholesterol, or bone density).
    - If there is an issue, at least you can address it head-on. If not, you can continue your normal routine with more peace of mind.

Sticking to a pattern of routine check-ups is a proactive step. You do not have to wait until you feel unwell to see a healthcare professional. Instead, you show up on your own terms, ready to learn about your body and keep it in better shape.

Key Elements of a Typical Check-Up

1. **Physical Examination**
    - The doctor or nurse often begins by checking your weight, height, and temperature. They may also measure blood pressure and heart rate.
    - Listening to your heart and lungs with a stethoscope can reveal signs like irregular beats or breathing patterns that need attention.
2. **Medical History Update**
    - Your provider might ask about any changes since your last visit. This includes new pains, shifts in energy level, or updates in your family's health history.
    - Keeping a small notebook can help you remember details to share, like certain days you felt more tired or any side effects from medications.
3. **Medication Review**

- Many older adults have multiple prescriptions. During a check-up, the doctor confirms you are still on the right doses and that the drugs do not conflict with one another.
    - Over-the-counter supplements or herbal products can matter too. It is best to mention everything you take, so the provider has a clear picture.
4. **Suggestions for Further Tests**
    - If the doctor notices something that needs more study, they may refer you for imaging (like X-rays or scans) or ask for bloodwork.
    - This step helps them gather more info if a certain result seems off or if you are at a higher risk for a specific issue.
5. **Time for Questions**
    - A good check-up includes open dialogue. You can ask, "Is my blood pressure okay?" or "What about my risk for certain conditions?"
    - If instructions for new medication or screenings feel complicated, ask for clearer explanations or written notes.

These basics often fit into one appointment. Depending on your health, some check-ups will be brief, while others might need more discussion or multiple visits.

Common Screenings for Older Adults

1. **Blood Pressure Checks**
    - This is one of the simplest and most frequent screenings. If pressure is too high, it can stress the heart and blood vessels.
    - Controlling high blood pressure may involve medication or small shifts in daily habits. Catching it early can help reduce the risk of serious heart issues.
2. **Cholesterol and Lipid Tests**
    - A blood test can measure levels of "bad" (LDL) and "good" (HDL) cholesterol, as well as triglycerides.
    - High LDL cholesterol might suggest an increased chance of clogged arteries, which can lead to heart attacks or strokes. If results are high, doctors may recommend medication or changes in eating habits.
3. **Blood Sugar (Diabetes) Screening**

- Another blood test, called fasting blood glucose or A1C, checks if sugar levels are elevated.
- If the test shows prediabetes or diabetes, early steps, such as medication or certain meal plans, can help avoid complications that might affect the eyes, kidneys, or nerves.

4. **Colon Cancer Screening**
   - As people age, the risk of colon cancer can rise. Various screening options include colonoscopy, stool tests, or sigmoidoscopy.
   - Colonoscopies help doctors see the entire colon, find and remove small growths (polyps) before they can turn cancerous.

5. **Breast Cancer Screening (for Women)**
   - Mammograms are X-rays of breast tissue that can find tumors that are too small to feel. Regular screening guidelines differ by age and health status, but older women may continue mammograms based on doctor advice.

6. **Prostate Cancer Screening (for Men)**
   - Some men choose blood tests (PSA) or exams to check for prostate changes. Not everyone needs it, and doctors often weigh risks and benefits with the patient.
   - Talk with a healthcare provider to see if this test fits your situation.

7. **Bone Density Tests**
   - A DEXA scan measures bone thickness (bone mineral density). Thinner bones can lead to fractures or osteoporosis.
   - Finding low bone density early may lead to treatments that bolster bones, like certain medications or supplements.

8. **Eye and Ear Checks**
   - We have touched on eye and ear care in a previous chapter, but screenings with specialists can detect glaucoma, cataracts, or hearing decline before they get too advanced.
   - Regular visits to an eye doctor or hearing professional might be advised if you notice changes.

These are just a few examples of recommended screenings. The exact timeline varies by person. Some tests might happen every year, while others occur every few years or only once you reach a certain age.

Preparing for a Check-Up

1. **Gather Personal Information**
   - Have a list of all medications (including dose and frequency), over-the-counter pills, and any herbs or vitamins you use.
   - Note any recent changes in appetite, sleep patterns, or pain. Summaries can help you recall details once in the exam room.
2. **Plan Your Questions**
   - If you have specific issues—like a rash that appears on your arm every week—write them down so you will remember to mention them.
   - Bring a friend or family member if you feel you might forget details from the conversation.
3. **Check for Instructions**
   - Some tests need special prep. For instance, you might need to fast before a blood sugar or cholesterol check.
   - If you are not sure about what is required, call the clinic ahead of time.
4. **Comfortable Clothing**
   - Wear clothes that are easy to remove or roll up in case the doctor needs to check certain areas or measure blood pressure on the upper arm.
   - If you use a walker or cane, let the staff know. They can make sure the exam room is set for safety.
5. **Bring Health Documents**
   - If you have results from past procedures or a summary of medical visits from a different provider, carrying them to the next check-up can save time and reduce confusion.
   - This is especially useful if you have changed doctors or moved to a new area.

Being prepared can turn a doctor's visit from a rushed event into a calmer discussion where you can share and learn effectively.

Communicating with Healthcare Providers

1. **Being Honest**
   - It is important to speak frankly about any symptoms or concerns, even if they feel embarrassing. Doctors have heard many issues before and appreciate accurate info.

- If you have not followed a past suggestion or if you stopped taking a medicine, let them know. Hiding this can lead to confusion or incorrect treatments.
2. **Asking for Explanations**
    - Doctors might use medical words you do not recognize. It is perfectly okay to say, "Can you please explain that more simply?"
    - A good provider will clarify in plain language, ensuring you understand your situation.
3. **Taking Notes**
    - Jotting down key points—like medication changes or follow-up steps—can keep you on track after you leave the office.
    - If you are not a strong note-taker, ask a friend or relative to attend and help remember the details.
4. **Follow-Up Questions**
    - If you go home and realize something is unclear, do not hesitate to call the clinic. A nurse or receptionist can often pass your question to the provider or schedule another time to discuss.
    - Good communication extends beyond the face-to-face appointment.

The doctor-patient relationship works best as a partnership. You are the one living with your body every day, and the doctor brings medical knowledge. Together, you can make better decisions.

Overcoming Fear or Anxiety About Screenings

1. **Understanding the Purpose**
    - Sometimes, people avoid screenings because they fear bad news. However, ignoring possible problems does not make them go away.
    - Realizing that these tests are designed to protect or help you, not to cause alarm, can shift your mindset.
2. **Asking About Discomfort**
    - Certain exams, like a colonoscopy, might seem scary. Asking the provider about how they manage comfort, sedation, and how long it takes can ease worries.
    - Many screening tools have become less invasive over time, with sedation or new technologies that reduce pain.
3. **Small Steps**

- If you are nervous about multiple tests, talk to the doctor about spacing them out.
- Handling them one at a time might feel more manageable than doing everything at once.
4. **Support from Loved Ones**
    - If a friend or relative has gone through the same screening, hearing their experience may help.
    - You can also bring someone along for emotional support if the test is done in a clinic.

Facing a screening can be easier when you remember it is part of caring for yourself. Whether you receive a clean bill of health or discover a concern, you have more control over the outcome by knowing what is going on in your body.

What Happens After Screenings

1. **Test Results**
    - Some results come quickly (like a blood pressure reading), while others, like a lab test for cholesterol, might take a few days.
    - Ask how you will receive the results: a phone call, a follow-up visit, or an online system. If you do not hear back, reach out.
2. **Interpreting Numbers**
    - Lab results might show certain ranges—for example, normal, borderline, or high. The doctor can explain if a result is okay for you and if any next steps are needed.
    - Even if a value is out of range, it may not always be serious, but it is worth a conversation on what to do next.
3. **Further Testing or Treatment**
    - Some screenings lead to more tests. For instance, if a colonoscopy finds a polyp, it might be removed or tested.
    - If a mammogram looks unusual, a follow-up imaging test might be scheduled. This does not always mean cancer; it could be a routine check to clarify a shadow.
4. **Lifestyle or Medication Tweaks**
    - Depending on results, you might be asked to try a new medication, adjust a current dose, or keep a closer eye on certain symptoms.
    - Even a slight shift—such as checking blood pressure at home more often—can make a difference.

The important part is not to panic if you see an odd result. Most of the time, doctors have ways to handle or watch these changes. Regular check-ups are all about being proactive.

Speciality Check-Ups

1. **Dermatology**
    - A skin specialist might look for suspicious moles, unusual rashes, or early signs of skin cancer. Older adults often have more spots or dryness, so a professional check can be reassuring.
    - If you have a mole that changed shape or color, mentioning it quickly to a dermatologist can catch problems early.
2. **Orthopedic or Bone Specialist**
    - If bone density is low, or if you have ongoing joint issues, a specialist might suggest certain therapies, injections, or supportive devices.
    - These measures can lessen pain and reduce the chance of fractures.
3. **Cardiology**
    - If your doctor hears an irregular heartbeat or you have a family history of heart trouble, a cardiologist might check you further.
    - This can involve an EKG, stress test, or other specialized scans to ensure your heart is functioning well.
4. **Neurology**
    - Memory changes or unusual headaches might lead to an evaluation by a neurologist, who can test for things like mild cognitive concerns or nerve problems.
    - Early diagnosis can offer more strategies to remain as sharp and independent as possible.

Seeing specialists might feel like a hassle, but they bring expert insight. If your primary doctor recommends it, it usually means the issue is specific enough to need closer attention.

Costs and Coverage

1. **Insurance Plans**

- Some screenings are covered by certain insurance plans, especially if they are recommended at a national level.
- Check your plan or ask the clinic which screenings are fully paid for and which might have additional charges.

2. **Annual Wellness Programs**
    - In some places, older adults have access to yearly wellness checks at no cost.
    - Taking advantage of these can save money and keep you on top of basic health measures.
3. **Sliding Scale Clinics**
    - If insurance is limited, certain clinics use a sliding scale based on income.
    - This can help manage costs for important tests, ensuring finances do not block you from needed screenings.
4. **Asking Questions About Bills**
    - Do not be shy about contacting your insurance provider or the doctor's office about potential fees.
    - If money is tight, let the medical team know. They might find ways to reduce costs or suggest alternative testing that is more budget-friendly.

Financial worries should not keep older adults from check-ups that can prevent bigger bills later. Sometimes, an early fix is cheaper and safer than treating an advanced condition.

When to Seek Urgent Assessment

1. **Sudden Changes**
    - If you experience fast-onset symptoms like severe chest pain, confusion, or extreme dizziness, a regular check-up is not enough. You might need emergency care.
    - Seeking help quickly can limit damage and improve the chance of a good outcome.
2. **High Fever or Continuous Vomiting**
    - If you cannot keep fluids down or if a fever persists, it is better to call a healthcare provider or go to urgent care.
    - Older adults can become dehydrated more easily, so prompt action is vital.

3. **Pain That Grows**
    - Gradual, mild pain can wait until the next appointment. But pain that intensifies or disrupts daily tasks might need immediate evaluation.
    - This is especially true for back pain that includes numbness in the legs or trouble walking.
4. **Bleeding or Discharge**
    - Unexpected bleeding, such as blood in the urine or stool, calls for prompt checks. It might be a simple cause, but ignoring it could lead to larger concerns.
    - The same goes for unusual discharge from the eyes, ears, or any wound.

Routine screenings are for normal, scheduled health checks. Urgent signs cannot wait. Knowing the difference can save you from serious complications.

Maintaining a Personal Health Record

1. **Tracking Results**
    - Keep a folder with copies of lab results, imaging reports, and immunization records.
    - Some older adults find it useful to note their normal ranges—like what is a typical cholesterol or blood pressure reading for them.
2. **Medication Updates**
    - If the doctor changes a prescription, mark it in your record with the date and reason.
    - Keeping a current list is handy if you see a new specialist or wind up in an emergency room.
3. **Appointment Dates**
    - You can write down each visit's date, the main focus, and any changes recommended.
    - This record acts like a quick timeline of your health journey, making it simpler to remember how things developed.
4. **Accessible Location**
    - Store these health papers in a safe but easy-to-reach spot at home, so you (or a family member) can grab them quickly in case of an unexpected hospital trip.
    - Some people also keep digital copies in password-protected files.

A personal health record can reduce confusion between different doctors and empower you to see the big picture of your well-being.

Coordinating with Other Providers

1. **Multiple Specialists**
   - If you see different specialists—like a cardiologist, dermatologist, or neurologist—ensure they each know what the others have found or prescribed.
   - Your primary care doctor can help gather all the details, but you can also share your personal record if needed.
2. **Pharmacy Alerts**
   - Some pharmacies can flag potential drug interactions when you fill prescriptions.
   - Always use the same pharmacy if possible, so they have a full record of your medications.
3. **Home Health and Caregivers**
   - If you receive home health visits, let them know about upcoming screenings or follow-up appointments.
   - Caregivers can assist you in preparing for tests and ensuring you follow any pre-visit instructions.
4. **Communication Tools**
   - Some medical systems have online portals where you can email doctors or view test results. If technology is challenging, ask for a tutorial or get a family member to guide you.
   - Alternatively, phone calls remain a reliable method for older adults who are less comfortable online.

Keeping everything coordinated helps avoid repeated tests, missed instructions, or medication conflicts. It also helps you feel more confident in your plan.

CHAPTER 20: CREATING A SAFE AND COMFORTABLE HOME

Home should be a place of comfort, calmness, and safety. For older adults, the home environment can either support daily routines or create hurdles that lead to stress, falls, or injuries. As the years go by, certain changes—like reduced balance or vision—may make a once-comfortable house tricky to navigate. Fortunately, many low-cost or simple adjustments can improve safety and ease. In this final chapter, we will explore practical ways to transform your living space into a secure, convenient place that encourages confidence. We will avoid repeating earlier details about stress or social connections, focusing instead on the physical environment and everyday tasks that can be simplified with thoughtful design.

Why Home Safety Matters More in Later Years

1. **Changing Abilities**
    - Even if you feel strong, small shifts in reaction time or depth perception can impact your movements around the house.
    - Reducing potential hazards can help prevent minor stumbles or bigger accidents.
2. **Desire for Independence**
    - Many older adults want to live on their own terms, without depending too much on family or care facilities.
    - A safe home environment can extend the time a person can remain independent, performing daily activities with minimal outside help.
3. **Peace of Mind**
    - Worrying about tripping over loose rugs or struggling to reach items on high shelves can add mental strain.
    - Removing dangers and adding supportive features can lower these worries, letting you focus on more pleasant things.
4. **Cost Savings**
    - Falls and accidents can lead to hospital bills or the need for in-home nursing afterward.

- Spending a bit of effort now to add rails or improve lighting might cost far less than dealing with medical bills from a preventable injury.

Addressing home safety does not mean giving up style or personal taste. Often, it is about small tweaks or reorganizing things so they are more suitable for the current stage of life.

Entryways and Door Areas

1. **Well-Lit Entrance**
   - A bright porch light can help you see steps or doormats clearly, especially at night or in dim weather.
   - Motion-sensor lights can turn on automatically when you approach, reducing the need to fumble for switches.
2. **Stable Door Handles**
   - Handles that are easy to grip (such as lever-style handles instead of round knobs) can make opening doors simpler if you have arthritis or reduced hand strength.
   - Ensure the door lock is not too high or tough to operate. Some people choose electronic keypads that remove the need for keys.
3. **Clear Pathways**
   - If your front steps have cracks or uneven patches, consider repairs or installing a small ramp.
   - Keep the walkway free of clutter like pots or decorations. This prevents tripping when carrying groceries or if you need a walker.
4. **Door Thresholds**
   - A high threshold or metal strip can catch toes or canes. If possible, have it reduced or replaced with a low-profile version.
   - Some older adults add a small transition ramp if the threshold is too tall to remove.

Making it easy and safe to enter and exit the home is a major first step. The entryway sets the tone for comfort in the rest of the house.

Living Room and Common Areas

1. **Open Floor Space**
   - Cluttered or tight furniture arrangements can block walking paths. Keeping a clear route from the couch to the door or to other rooms helps reduce falls.
   - If an older coffee table has sharp corners, adding corner guards can lessen the chance of bruises if bumped.
2. **Stable Furniture**
   - Chairs and couches that are too low or soft can be hard to get up from. Consider chairs with firm seats and armrests for support.
   - Wobbly side tables or lamps can topple if leaned on. Checking them and tightening screws can improve stability.
3. **Non-Slip Rugs or Mats**
   - Throw rugs can be a major hazard if they move or curl at the edges. If you love rugs, use non-slip backings or tape them down so they stay flat.
   - Alternatively, removing loose rugs entirely might be the safest solution if you have concerns about tripping.
4. **Adequate Lighting**
   - Good lighting is crucial, especially near corners or stair landings. Table lamps should be easy to switch on without stretching.
   - If overhead lights are not bright enough, adding floor lamps in dim corners can help you see better, reducing the risk of bumping into furniture.

A living area that is free of hazards and well-lit can act as a welcoming spot for relaxation, reading, or chatting with visitors.

Kitchen Adjustments

1. **Easy-Access Cabinets**
   - Storing frequently used items—like plates, cups, and pans—within comfortable reach reduces stretching or climbing on stools.
   - If some shelves are too high, a sturdy step stool with a handle can help, but it is best to keep daily items at waist or shoulder level.
2. **Organizing Countertops**

        - Keep counters clear of random gadgets. This leaves space for safe food prep and lessens the chance of knocking things off.
        - A small container to gather cooking utensils can help you avoid digging in drawers for needed tools.
    3. **Appliance Safety**
        - Check cords for wear or fraying. If an appliance is old or acts oddly, replacing it might be safer.
        - Stove controls at the front or side are easier to reach than those at the back, reducing the need to reach over hot burners. If your stove has back knobs, be extra careful or consider shifting to a safer model.
    4. **Non-Skid Floor Mats**
        - A mat in front of the sink can provide comfort for feet if you stand there often. Ensure it has a non-skid bottom.
        - Spills are inevitable while cooking. Wipe them up promptly so the floor does not become slick.

The kitchen is a busy zone. By placing items in logical spots and ensuring stable footing, you can enjoy cooking or snack prep with more confidence and fewer accidents.

Bedroom Comfort and Safety

1. **Bed Height**
    - A bed that is too low or too high can be troublesome to get in or out of. Adjusting bed frame height or adding a firm mattress can assist you in standing up more easily.
    - Some older adults use bed rails or attach a grip handle to the side for extra support.
2. **Clear Path to the Bathroom**
    - Many older adults wake at night to use the bathroom. Keeping a direct route free of clothes, shoes, or boxes reduces the risk of tripping when sleepy.
    - A small nightlight with a gentle glow can guide you without blinding brightness.
3. **Nearby Essentials**

- A bedside table with a lamp, glass of water, tissues, and perhaps a phone can be helpful. This way, you do not have to stretch or walk around if you need something in the middle of the night.
- For emergencies, having a phone close at hand (or a call button if you live alone and have health concerns) is wise.

4. **Temperature Control**
    - Some older adults feel cold easily at night or might sweat more. Keep soft blankets that are easy to remove or add.
    - A fan, air conditioner, or space heater should be used carefully to avoid overheating or fire hazards. Make sure the cords are away from walkways.

A bedroom that supports restful sleep and easy nighttime movement can help reduce falls, improve mood, and encourage better rest.

Bathroom Adjustments

1. **Grab Bars and Handrails**
    - Wet surfaces are slippery. Installing grab bars near the toilet and in the shower or tub can provide stable holds.
    - Towel bars are not strong enough to act as grab bars, so specialized fixtures must be used. They are made to hold body weight without coming loose.
2. **Non-Slip Mats**
    - A bath mat with rubber backing inside the tub or shower can stop feet from sliding.
    - Outside, another absorbent mat prevents water from creating a slick floor.
3. **Raised Toilet Seat**
    - If sitting down or standing up from the toilet is challenging, a raised seat or a commode chair can ease the strain on knees and hips.
    - Some designs include built-in handrails on the side for added support.
4. **Shower Chairs or Benches**
    - Standing for the entire shower can feel unsteady. A waterproof bench or seat gives you a place to sit while washing.

- Handheld showerheads are also helpful, letting you direct the water flow wherever needed while seated.

The bathroom is often the spot of greatest concern for slips. But a few well-placed bars, mats, and seat options can transform it into a safer space.

Lighting and Electrical Concerns

1. **Light Switches**
   - Switches that glow faintly in the dark can be easier to find at night.
   - Installing switches at both ends of a hallway or near each door can help you turn lights on before entering a dark area.
2. **Nightlights in Hallways**
   - Plugging in a small nightlight with a sensor can keep walkways lit if you need to move around at odd hours.
   - This is especially important near stairs or corners where you might not expect a step.
3. **Power Cords and Outlets**
   - Loose cords stretched across the floor can trip you. If possible, route them behind furniture or along walls using clips or cord covers.
   - Avoid overloading outlets with many plugs. Using a surge protector or power strip with a built-in circuit breaker can be safer.
4. **Battery-Powered Lights**
   - In case of power outages, keep a flashlight or battery-powered lantern handy.
   - Make sure batteries are fresh or replaced regularly so you are not left in the dark during an emergency.

Proper lighting helps older adults move confidently, while careful attention to electrical safety lowers the risk of shocks or fire.

Stairs and Hallways

1. **Sturdy Handrails**
    - Both sides of a staircase can benefit from handrails. Having support for either hand can make going up and down much safer.
    - If the existing rail is shaky, reinforce or replace it. It needs to hold your weight if you slip.
2. **Non-Slip Treads**
    - If stairs are wooden or smooth, consider adding non-slip strips or carpet runners so your feet have better grip.
    - Avoid fancy patterns that can camouflage edges. A clear contrast between step edges helps you see where to place your foot.
3. **Good Lighting Over Steps**
    - A bright overhead fixture or step lights can show each step clearly. If a hallway is dim, it is easy to misjudge stair height.
    - If you have a landing or turn in the stairs, ensure that corner has a separate light or a well-placed fixture.
4. **Considering a Stair Lift**
    - If climbing stairs is too demanding or risky, some older adults install a stair lift—an electric seat that glides along a track on the stairway.
    - While these can be more expensive, they allow continued use of upstairs rooms without constant fear of falling.

Stairs do not have to force you out of your home if you can secure them or adapt them with the right aids.

Outdoor Spaces and Yards

1. **Even Walkways**
    - A cracked sidewalk or an uneven patio stone is easy to trip on. Fixing these hazards or leveling them can cut down on stumbles.
    - If you have a garden path with gravel or stepping stones, ensure they are stable and not prone to shifting.
2. **Railings on Outdoor Steps**
    - Just like indoor stairs, outdoor steps to a porch or deck should have sturdy railings.

- If you live in a climate with snow or ice, consider a rough surface paint or slip-resistant treads for steps.
3. **Accessible Gardening**
    - If you enjoy gardening, raised beds can let you work without bending all the way to the ground. This can protect your back and knees.
    - Tools with extended handles or lightweight designs can make yard work easier on wrists and shoulders.
4. **Safe Lighting Outside**
    - Path lights or solar-powered stakes can illuminate walkways at night, preventing missteps.
    - Make sure your mailbox area or trash bins are also reachable without stepping in dark patches or uneven ground.

Even if you love spending time outside, ensuring the yard is free of hidden dangers keeps you active and happy with fewer injuries.

Technology Aids and Smart Devices

1. **Emergency Call Systems**
    - Devices worn as a pendant or wristband can let you push a button to call for help if you fall or cannot reach a phone. Some even detect a fall automatically.
    - If living alone, this can bring peace of mind, knowing that help is just a button press away.
2. **Smart Home Devices**
    - Voice-activated assistants can turn on lights or make calls without you having to move. This can be handy if you feel unsteady or your hands are busy.
    - Smart doorbells with cameras let you see who is at the door before you answer, improving security.
3. **Motion Sensors**
    - Lights that turn on automatically when you enter a room or hallway can eliminate fumbling for switches.
    - Sensor-activated faucets might help if turning handles is hard on your wrists.
4. **Medication Reminders**

- Electronic pill dispensers beep when it is time for a dose, preventing missed or double doses.
- Some apps on smartphones can also alert you, but a dedicated dispenser can be simpler if you prefer not to handle complex gadgets.

Technology can play a helpful role in home safety, but choosing devices that fit your comfort level is key. Overly complex systems might be frustrating if you are not used to them.

Emergency Preparedness

1. **Phone Accessibility**
    - Keep a phone close by, especially if you have mobility issues. In many households, cordless phones or cell phones are the norm, but ensure they are charged and within easy reach.
    - Storing emergency numbers in speed dial (like 911, a neighbor, or close family) can save time under stress.
2. **Fire Safety**
    - Working smoke detectors and a simple fire extinguisher in the kitchen are essential. Test alarms regularly to confirm the batteries are fresh.
    - Plan how you would exit if a fire breaks out. If you have difficulty with stairs, consider living on a floor with a safe exit path.
3. **Carbon Monoxide Detectors**
    - If you use gas heaters or appliances, a carbon monoxide detector can warn you of invisible fumes.
    - Place it near bedrooms so it can wake you if levels rise while you sleep.
4. **Escape Routes and Contacts**
    - In multi-story homes, keep in mind how you would get down safely if the main stairs are blocked. Some people store a collapsible ladder near a window.
    - Have a small bag with important documents or medication lists if you need to leave quickly for a weather emergency or other crisis.

Planning for emergencies can feel daunting, but it is another way to remain in control. The hope is that you never need these measures, yet they are there if something happens.

Balancing Safety with Comfort

1. **Maintaining Personal Style**
   - Installing grab bars or simpler door handles does not mean your home must feel like a hospital. Many home improvement stores sell stylish, sturdy options that fit your aesthetic.
   - Colors, fabrics, and personal decorations can still flourish. Just ensure that safety is woven into the design.
2. **Focusing on Ease of Use**
   - Items you use daily—like remote controls, reading glasses, or books—should be stored where you can get them without bending or stretching too far.
   - If you like crafts or puzzles, set up a stable table with good lighting to avoid eye strain or uncomfortable postures.
3. **Gradual Changes**
   - You do not have to redo the entire house at once. Start with the areas that pose the biggest risk (like the bathroom or stairs) and address others step by step.
   - Over time, small upgrades can add up to a significantly safer environment.
4. **Testing New Ideas**
   - If you are unsure about a rearrangement, try it for a week. For instance, moving a chair or a lamp to a different spot might make the flow better.
   - You can always tweak the layout again. It is an ongoing process.

The goal is to enjoy a home that is both protective and welcoming. Simple changes can keep you feeling at ease without turning your space into something unrecognizable.

When Extra Help Is Needed

1. **Home Health Services**
   - For those recovering from surgery or dealing with ongoing conditions, a visiting nurse or therapist might guide further home modifications.
   - They can spot hazards, suggest ways to manage tasks, or help with medication organization.

2. **Professional Assessments**
   - Some agencies provide free or low-cost home safety evaluations for older adults. Professionals walk through the house and point out risks or solutions.
   - Occupational therapists can tailor suggestions based on specific health conditions, ensuring you have the right tools for daily tasks.
3. **Hiring a Handyperson**
   - If installing grab bars or adjusting rails feels too complex, a handyman or carpenter can do it properly.
   - Ensuring it is done right can save money over the long term and offer greater stability.
4. **Considering a Downsized or Assisted Option**
   - If the house remains too big to manage, or if many repairs are needed, some older adults move to smaller apartments or senior living communities.
   - In such settings, certain safety features are often built-in, and staff is available if something goes wrong.

Recognizing when you need more support is a sign of wisdom, not weakness. The aim is to stay as active as possible in a home that fits your current abilities and preferences.

Closing Thoughts: A Home for Well-Being

- **Personalizing Safety**: Each person has unique needs. Some older adults might need stronger lighting due to lower vision, while others need more robust railings because of balance concerns.
- **Small Tweaks, Big Benefits**: Replacing round doorknobs with lever handles or adding a simple shower chair can drastically lower the chance of an accident.
- **Staying Active**: A safe home encourages movement. If the environment feels risky, older adults might stay seated too much out of fear. Removing that fear can inspire healthier daily living.
- **Adapting Over Time**: As you age, revisit your home setup. What works now might need adjusting in a few years. Keeping up with changes ensures ongoing comfort.
- **Team Effort**: Relatives, friends, or professional services can all pitch in to identify areas for improvement. Even a quick chat with a neighbor could lead to a suggestion about better lighting or slip-resistant floors.

Your home is a reflection of your life experiences and personal tastes. By taking steps to make it safer, you uphold both comfort and independence. Whether you choose minor fixes, major renovations, or eventually consider a different place to live, the core goal stays the same: enjoying a space that lets you go through daily tasks with confidence, fosters a sense of calmness, and fits your physical and emotional needs. With these adjustments, your home can remain a steady foundation for well-being as you move through later life with greater assurance.

Printed in Great Britain
by Amazon